Malaria

Margaret Humphreys

# Malaria
*Poverty, Race, and*
*Public Health*
*in the United States*

The
Johns Hopkins
University
Press
*Baltimore*
*and London*

© 2001 The Johns Hopkins University Press
All rights reserved. Published 2001
Printed in the United States of America on acid-free paper
9 8 7 6 5 4 3 2 1

The Johns Hopkins University Press
2715 North Charles Street
Baltimore, Maryland 21218-4363
www.press.jhu.edu

Library of Congress Cataloging-in-Publication Data
Humphreys, Margaret, 1955–
    Malaria: poverty, race, and public health
in the United States / Margaret Humphreys.
        p. cm.
Includes bibliographical references and index.
ISBN 0-8018-6637-5
1. Malaria—United States—History.  I. Title.
RC161.A2 H86 2001
616.9′362′00973—dc21          00-011292

A catalog record for this book is available from the British Library.

For Ted

# Contents

# Acknowledgments

Like most historians who compose such essays, I have been continually amazed at how cheerfully others have lent their time and effort to my research project. In the eight years that have seen this book to completion, I have accrued many debts, and it is a privilege to be able to acknowledge them here. Without the institutional support of Duke University, it is unlikely that this book would have been written. The opportunity to come here in 1993 with a joint appointment in medicine and history liberated me from full-time medical practice and administration, allowing time once again for historical research and writing. Over the ensuing years Duke has supported this project in ways large and small, with sabbaticals, small travel grants for archive work and meetings, research assistants, office space, modern computers, ample libraries, a photocopying budget, and the all-important peace of tenure. I am grateful to the department chairs and deans, especially Alex Roland, William Chafe, and Richard White, who helped make all that possible.

The most important institutional contribution has been, of course, the presence of exciting and supportive colleagues. Several have read the manuscript in full—Peter English, John Herd Thompson, and John W. Cell—and they have made this a much better book. Seymour Mauskopf, Michael McVaugh, and Keith Wailoo have commented on the project at various stages, and generally been invaluable for their friendship and support. Other colleagues, especially Kristen Neuschel, Jean O'Barr, Anne Firor Scott, Kate Joyce, Jehanne Gheith, Wendy Wall, Ron Witt, Peter Wood, Jan Ewald, Ed Balleisen, David Barry Gaspar, and Kären Wigen have contributed by making my intellectual and social life at Duke joyous and fulfilling.

Every scholar hopes that they are writing for an interested and enlightened audience and takes succor from the knowledge that such an audience actually exists. I've mainly found my audience at meetings of the American Association for the History of Medicine and have benefited from many hallway conversations and questions at sessions over the years. Although my direct intellectual debt is noted where relevant in the footnotes, the influence of other scholars is here in many indirect ways, and they deserve thanks: Caroline Hannaway, Victoria Harden, Charles Rosenberg, Barbara Rosenkrantz, Kenneth Ludmerer, Joel Howell, John Eyler, Gerry Grob, Günter Risse, Norman Gevitz, John Parascandola, Suzanne White Junod, John Harley Warner, Naomi Rogers, Russell Maulitz, Molly Sutphen, Ellen More, Judith Walzer Leavitt, Robert Joy, Dale Smith, Susan Lederer, and Jacalyn Duffin. Papers that evolved from this project were presented at Johns Hopkins, the University of Michigan, University of California at San Francisco, the Wellcome Institute, the University of North Carolina at Chapel Hill, Yale University, New York University, the University of Toronto, and East Carolina University, as well as at AAHM meetings, the Society for the Social History of Medicine, and the Southeast Regional Mosquito Control Association. I am grateful to all for the feedback, questions, and comments I received in these venues. Perhaps my most valued comment came from Philip Curtin after a contentious seminar presentation at Johns Hopkins on the core argument of the book; he said, simply, that he thought I was right.

There is a community of international scholars with an interest in the history of malaria who have met several times over the last decade. I was fortunate to attend two meetings of this group, the International Network for the History of Malaria, one in Annecy, France, in 1996 and the other at the Rockefeller Archive Center in North Tarrytown, New York, in 1998. My knowledge of the history of malaria expanded enormously at these two sessions, and I'd particularly like to thank Bill Bynum, Mary Dobson, Randall Packard, Peter Brown, Socrates Litsios, Mary Malowany, Anne-Emanuelle Birn, and Wolfgang Eckart for their contributions.

Archivists and librarians are central to the historian's task, and several have helped me along the way. Suzanne Porter, the librarian of the Duke medical history collection, has located microforms, found obscure volumes, and otherwise offered assistance throughout the project. At the CDC archives in East Point, Georgia, Mary Ann Hawkins was persistently cheerful as we struggled together through box after box of poorly labeled material. Barry Engber, the medical entomologist of the state of North Carolina, doesn't quite count as an archivist, but he did contact me about materials his office had in storage that related to the malaria campaigns of the 1930s and 1940s. He gave me a desk to work at, free photocopying, and full access to the boxes of material he had found stored in an old barn. Darwin Stapleton, the director of the Rockefeller Archive Center, is a historian of malaria himself and hence doubly valuable as a guide to the relevant materials in the Rockefeller collection that pertain to malaria. He and his staff were consistently gracious and patient with demands for multiple boxes in minimal time.

A Burroughs-Wellcome Medical History Research Grant provided much-needed sabbatical time. The Josiah Charles Trent Memorial Foundation provided travel grants for archival work and also funds for the purchase of research materials and equipment.

Two essays have appeared in print that are drawn from this project, and I am grateful for permission to reproduce revised versions of that material here. Text on malaria control projects in the 1930s (chapter 5) appeared in a similar form in "Water Won't Run Uphill: The New Deal and Malaria Control in the American South, 1933–1940," *Parassitologia* 40 (1998): 183–91. The 1940s DDT campaigns (Chapter 7) are described in "Kicking a Dying Dog: DDT and the Demise of Malaria in the American South, 1942–1950," *Isis* 87 (1996): 1–17.

My friend Ann Brown kept me focused on the important things in life, like dogs, good food, and the beach, when this project threatened to become too overwhelming. My parents, Mary and K. B. Humphreys, have offered continual support, and my mother read the manuscript from end to end, applying her English teacher's red pencil to much of my prose.

Finally, I come to Ted Kerin. He has made a modest direct impact on the book, mainly as a supplier of patent medicine advertisements found through dogged persistence on the Internet. He came back into my life only during the last year or so of the book's construction, but he has totally transformed my existence, bringing me happiness and contentment that I never knew were possible. It gives me great joy to dedicate this book to him.

# Introduction

"Has Malaria Disappeared?" one hopeful southern medical editor asked at midcentury. "Malaria Reduced to the Vanishing Point," proclaimed the U.S. Public Health Service in jubilant answer.[1] American malariologists had good reason for breaking open the champagne in 1950. Malaria, a disease that had plagued the country from its earliest years as a colony, was gone. Passed from person to person by the bite of the female anopheles mosquito, malaria parasites cause debilitating fevers and sometimes death. Malaria was a significant disease in American history, one that shaped southern and western history in particular through its impact on labor patterns, mortality rates, and settlement choices. Its demise was certainly cause for celebration.

Even though it is mostly a memory in the United States, malaria remains a major health disaster internationally. Malaria parasites killed millions of people during the 1990s, and sickened hundreds of times as many, and there is no prospect that these numbers will improve soon. As one international committee report put it, "The outlook for malaria control is grim. The disease . . . is present in 102 countries and is responsible for over 100 million clinical cases and 1–2 million deaths each year." Far from optimistic, the committee reported that the situation is growing worse, for "efforts to control malaria have met with less and less success."[2] This scourge has survived major international campaigns that were armed with insecticides against the vector and antibiotics against the parasite. Resistance to both weapons has emerged, and unless researchers create an effective vaccine, there is no hope on the horizon that malaria will retreat as a major world pestilence.

Most Americans think of malaria as a tropical nuisance, if they think of it at all. It is a problem for vacationers or missionaries or adopted children from foreign lands, not a part of their everyday lives. But malaria was once very much a prominent American disease, common in some areas as late as the 1940s. Cases are frequently imported into the United States today, which is not surprising since something like 40 percent of the world's population lives in malarious areas and international travel is so fluid and rapid.

Rarely, however, do new cases arise within the United States; imported parasites are usually contained within their host bodies. When indigenous (nonimported) cases do occur, it is headline news.[3] Malaria, once a painfully frequent presence in many parts of the United States, has become a tropical exotic. It has emerged as one of the diseases that separates the first, industrialized world from the third, developing sphere, or as some would have it, the "North" from the "South," globally conceived. The disappearance of malaria is one of the hallmarks of America's rise to world leadership, domination, and prosperity.

Why did malaria once flourish so readily in the United States, and why did it disappear? If it was a major plague on the nineteenth-century frontier, as it was, why is it a distinct anomaly in Omaha today? If there were well over a million cases of malaria in the South during the Great Depression, why were there fewer than a hundred in 1950? The first answer that comes to mind is that some combination of determined disease fighters and public health technology conquered malaria. But this is not what happened, either in the nineteenth century or in the twentieth. Accurate knowledge of the disease vector, the fact that mosquitoes spread malaria, was not at hand until 1897, so the retreat of malaria from the nineteenth-century frontier cannot be explained by deliberate public health action that specifically targeted the disease. And while the twentieth-century malaria picture was made much more complex by the existence of that etiological knowledge and measures based upon it, major socioeconomic factors, and not steps taken directly against parasite and vector, deserve the major credit for malaria's disappearance.

Most versions of malaria's career in the United States attribute its demise to the U.S. Public Health Service's DDT campaign of the 1940s. It is a plausible explanation, but at most it accounts for only a tiny percentage of malaria's reduction, since malaria had largely disappeared before it could be eradicated by DDT. DDT did finish off the last pockets of disease, but it cannot explain the rapid drop in malaria prevalence that occurred a few years before the spraying started. Understanding what brought about that drop means weighing the various prior public health efforts, aspects of lifestyle and poverty, and finally issues of geography. My solution to the mystery, tied heavily to geography and insect migration behavior, is supported but not proven by the evidence. The reader is warned that, like Robertson Davies's thematic puzzle, "Who killed Boy Staunton," you may be wiser at the end, but still not sure, about exactly "Who killed Malaria?"[4]

The history of malaria in the United States has given me a venue in which to develop multiple themes. One concerns the changing nature of public health work. Most nineteenth-century public health officials were physicians, although they cooperated with engineers in building sewers and drains. A simple board of health might have had physicians, a few concerned citizens, and perhaps an engineer. The twentieth-century public health enterprise involved multiple disciplines. Physicians were there, of course, but so were microscopists and other technicians, chemists, entomologists, pharmacologists, and engineers. Twentieth-century public health employees were largely full time as well, rather than the nineteenth-century model of the practicing physician who gave advice on public health matters as a sideline. Professionalism, characterized by specialism, had come to public health.

For the twentieth century, this story was dominated by a single theory of disease causation: malaria is caused by a plasmodium dispersed via mosquito bites. Gone were the nineteenth-century disputes over miasms, and quarrels over quarantine. Rather, the grand debate in the twentieth century was over the proper target of malaria control activity. Contending parties divided roughly into two camps: those who sought to kill the parasite within the human host, and those who sought to destroy the vector. Those who concentrated on the parasite went after it with drugs such as quinine and sometimes supported measures to increase human immunity through socioeconomic improvement. Attacking the vector could include spraying insecticides, draining wetlands to destroy mosquito breeding sites, and employing methods to separate humans from mosquitoes, such as screens and bednets. The controversy over the best malaria control method has yet to be resolved. Although apparent victories against malaria have been won in some countries, globally the disease flourishes. The "right" way to conquer malaria is still debated, making the ongoing discussions of this book's actors quite current today.[5]

In any history of malaria in the United States, race has to appear as a dominant topic. This is not just because of the innate immunities carried by some African-Americans, but also, and probably much more so, because the peculiar nexus of racism and poverty that has been the black's lot in the American South has created conditions ripe for malaria transmission. Throughout the book we will see that the African-American's situation directly affected malaria's course. In the first half of the twentieth century, when black people migrated to northern cities in increasing numbers, migration had a profound impact on the prevalence of malaria. When black sharecroppers gained some little power over their landlords because of the option of yearly movement, that could influence the likelihood of landlords to supply screens. On the other hand, their general powerlessness over housing quality and their lack of access to medicine and nutritious food encouraged malaria to thrive. The centrality of African-Americans to malaria's history depended both on their unique biological inheritance and on their peculiar social locus within the most tropical region of the United States.

An overriding concern of my prior work, *Yellow Fever and the South,* was to follow the economic basis of public health reform in the impoverished South during the last quarter of the nineteenth century.[6] In the case of yellow fever, the impetus for control came from merchants who were badly wounded by both disease and quarantine. The money for disease control programs largely came from outside the South, in the form of federal government appropriation, although a not inconsiderable sum was raised among affluent southerners themselves. State and local governments were generally too poor to pay for needed public works. The South certainly suffered no sudden burst of prosperity after yellow fever disappeared in 1905. If anything, the South was as poor in the 1920s and even poorer in the 1930s. In the case of malaria, money again came from outside, not just in federal monies but in foundation grants from the likes of the Rockefeller and Rosenwald Foundations, and the American Red Cross. Funds from the U.S. Public Health Service (USPHS) and its subsidiary, the CDC, were supplemented from state coffers as well as private philanthropy. Various New Deal programs had a direct and indirect effect on the South and the course of malaria. In addition, the underlying economic condition of the South did start to improve, especially during World War II. Thereafter funding was much more abundant, the agencies were entrenched and growing, and the federal government loomed even larger over the South. Following the money and the growth of government public health institutions is a steady thread of this narrative.

The chapters that follow tell the story of malaria's curious career in the United States. After examining the biology and evolution of the malaria parasite and its vector, Chapter 1 goes on to describe malaria's course in the American colonies. Chapter 2 takes the story into the nineteenth century, when malaria was the preeminent frontier disease, known by all to be caused by the evil emanations of swamps and other reservoirs of putrid vegetable matter. The century closed with a revolution in infectious disease etiology that revealed the unlikely fact that malaria was instead caused by a microorganism carried by a mosquito. In the twentieth century malaria retreated to the American South, and Chapter 3 explores the reasons for its persistence there, with a detailed discussion of importance of poverty, race, and geography in maintaining the disease. Chapters 4 and 5 describe the public health efforts launched against malaria in the South over the first four decades of the century. After detailing these initiatives, Chapter 5 concludes with an argument about one (and perhaps the only) major cause of malaria's decline in the late 1930s and early 1940s. The penultimate chapter explores attitudes toward health, disease, and malaria among lay southerners, contrasting their eclectic point of view with that of scientifically oriented public health professionals. Chapter 7 recounts the great DDT campaigns launched against malaria in the United States in the 1940s, and it contains the book's conclusion.

Writing the history of a disease is a fascinating but daunting task. This narrative will try to break down a complex story by considering it from three perspectives: those of the physician, the people, and the parasite. The term *medical* or *physician's* perspective implies the point of view held by physicians and other public health professionals, as reflected in medical journals and the records of public health agencies. This is by far the easiest perspective to research, since such abundant materials are available. The *people's* perspective is obviously much less uniform and harder to tease out, in part because it encompasses so many different perspectives. To say it is the viewpoint of the nonmedically trained is to include a group of people otherwise quite diverse. It lumps the sharecropper, planter, merchant, and legislator together; it clusters the young and the old, and people from different regions. And it is a notoriously difficult population to research. The higher the social class, the more available the records, even when the people themselves did not leave personal accounts. To some extent, their actions—passing public health legislation or paying for antimalarial measures—take the place of written testimony. The poorest of the poor traditionally leave no trace at all, and that would be the case here but for one by-product of Franklin Roosevelt's New Deal. The Federal Writers' Project interviewed hundreds of the South's poor rural population, giving a rare peek into their attitudes toward sickness, medicine, and malaria.

The *parasite's* "perspective" is the murkiest of all, leading us into the chancy field of historical epidemiology. Malaria has gone under many names in the past, and well into the twentieth century disease records in the United States are unreliable. We can track its faint path through personal accounts of symptoms, looking for disease descriptions that sound like malaria's striking chills and fever. In the twentieth century there were actual sightings, as microscopists began to routinely see the parasite and document its presence. Pursuing such historical epidemiology assumes that parasite and disease exist, that they are not mere social constructions of a certain place and time. This book considers it proven that the malaria parasite is spread by the anopheles mosquito, and that it causes the disease malaria. This is not to say that the disease did not carry different cultural meanings within different milieus, defined by time, geography, race, and class. Its diagnosis was often confused, especially with typhoid fever, and at times it is difficult for the historian to discern whether it was there at all. But underlying all that confusion were living organisms, the two sorts of malaria parasites predominant in the United States, and with effort we can at least begin to make out their paths.

These three perspectives on disease were never distinct from each other, a situation that requires the historian to follow not three separate lines but a maze of interlocking and shifting influences. Medical knowledge changed suddenly around 1900, as Alphonse Laveran's and Ronald Ross's work on the parasite and mosquito, respectively, emerged triumphant. The new etiological theory rapidly replaced the centuries-old knowledge that emanations from swamps, or bad air, caused malaria. *Replaced* is not quite the right word here, for the change happened at different rates in different communities. The medical community's ideas were transformed the most rapidly, but it still took over a decade for Laveran's work to be accepted. It is harder to pinpoint when the new ideas penetrated the general community. In Chapter 6 we will see that the old often stood next to the new, and that an eclectic mix of ideas rather than a given canon was the norm. And the young, learning about mosquitoes and malaria in school, might have ideas contrary to the adults in their families. The borders between traditional folk knowledge and modern medical knowledge were fuzzy and ill defined. The parasite, of course, had no thoughts at all but soon felt the impact of new vector-based control schemes.

I had once hoped that this research project might result in more than historical narrative, that it might actually bear relevance for the beleaguered international malaria community: What was it about the United States that led to malaria's conquest there? Could it be copied elsewhere? But the book contains no startling revelations about how to fight malaria. The reasons malaria declined within the United States were well known by the 1940s, although my emphasis on the various factors is my own and diverges from contemporary accounts. In retrospect, it is easy to predict that in global campaigns, DDT would fail and antimalarial drugs would develop resistance. Still, there are no simple measures discoverable from an earlier day to put in their place. Eradicating malaria in the United States was relatively easy, given modern technology, and malaria would be easy to conquer again here, should an outbreak appear. The United States is not a tropical country, its vectors are not particularly efficient, and its people, even the poorest, now have housing, food, and health care that provides the basics for protection from this disease. The history of malaria's disappearance from the United States has few lessons to offer for those struggling to combat the disease in its contemporary tropical homes.

One persistent regret is that my words cannot begin to give expression to all the pain and suffering that malaria brought to Americans during its rampages over the centuries. In spite of the material in Chapter 6, the voices of malaria's victims do not come through clearly enough here. Nor do the voices of their grieving parents, as malaria does particularly destroy children. For this endeavor, the novelist can sometimes best the historian. In Peter Matthiessen's novel about a missionary family named Quarrier who confront God and death in the jungles of South America, the couple's young son Billy lies dying of malaria. He made friends with the neighboring Indian children, and one Indian boy comes to him demanding that

Billy name the enemy that has brought this disease, so that his friends can take action against him. To the Indian boy, Billy's father says, "He has no enemy. He is very sick. He was made sick by the mosquito. His only enemy is the mosquito." After the children leave, Billy asks his passionately Christian father,

> "Why did God . . . You won't get mad at me?"
> "No, Bill, I won't get mad at you."
> "Then, why did God have to go and make mosquitoes?"
> "I don't know," Quarrier said. "I surely wish I knew."[7]

This narrative can only begin to sketch the meaning of malaria in the lives of millions of Americans over the course of their history.

## Chapter 1

The Pestilence
That Stalks
in Darkness

Malaria is an ancient disease, part of human experience from Neanderthal and Cro-Magnon times. It thrived on the shores of the Mediterranean Sea and it was described frequently in the writings of ancient Near Eastern, Greek, and Roman physicians. Perhaps malaria was one of the horrors from which the psalmist sought relief, proclaiming: "You will not fear the terror of the night, nor the arrow that flies by day, nor the pestilence that stalks in darkness nor the destruction that wastes at noonday."[1] The sense that disease lurked in the darkness was more than just superstition, for the malaria mosquito prefers to bite after sundown; cultural awareness of this pattern is reflected in the pervasive anxiety about disease-laden evening mists that appears throughout the world's literature. Writing the history of malaria in the United States requires grasping the continuity of the disease from ancient times, in lands occupied by humans far longer than the soil of the Western Hemisphere has been. Understanding this history involves first an awareness of the biology of malaria, its earliest evolution, and the association of race with patterns of malaria immunity.

### Biology of Malaria

Malaria is not a single disease in humans but is actually a family of four different diseases caused by four different parasites. The parasites are similar in appearance, all belonging to the genus *Plasmodia*. The four species names are *falciparum, vivax, malariae,* and *ovale*. The fevers caused by these four organisms vary enough in their clinical presentations that different labels evolved for their symptom complexes, even before microbiologists were able to distinguish them definitively around 1900. Yet their clinical syndromes overlap enough that their relationship to one another has been commonly recognized throughout recorded history. The historian can make fairly accurate guesses about which parasite is dominant in certain malaria outbreaks; at other times the presence of malaria at all is in question. The two dominant organisms in U.S. history were *falciparum* and *vivax,* and where appropriate their differences will be emphasized here, while at other times they will be lumped together into a combined malaria diagnosis. There was also *malariae* in North America, but when malariologists did parasite surveys in the twentieth century, looking at blood smears to identify particular organisms, it never showed up more than 1 percent of the time. *Malariae* acts much like *vivax,* and its presence as a specific species makes little impact on this story. *Ovale* does not occur outside of West Africa.[2]

*Falciparum* causes the most severe form of malaria. The victim suffers from intermittent high fevers, with a severe retro-orbital headache, parched throat, and diffuse body aches. The body can be wracked with abdominal cramping, diarrhea, and vomiting. Children, well only a few hours earlier, can go into frightening febrile seizures. The liver and spleen become enlarged, and if hepatic malfunction reaches a critical level, jaundice may follow. When the parasite reaches a high enough density in the body, it can cause deadly effects by clogging small arteries in the brain and kidneys, leading to loss of blood flow to essential areas. The resulting coma of cerebral malaria often presages death. Blood and protein in the urine of patients with renal malaria is also a dire sign. Mortality from *falciparum* malaria can range from 20 to 40 percent when untreated, especially in a host that has never seen the infection before and has no acquired immunity.

*Vivax* malaria causes a much more benign disease but a highly unpleasant one nonetheless. It can kill up to 5 percent of its victims, although usually mortality is much lower. Like *falciparum,* it causes a high fever, with skull-splitting headache and icy pains throughout the skeleton. As in all fever spikes, the body undergoes a change in the "thermostat" that regulates internal temperature. Sensing (falsely) that the body's temperature is too low, the hypothalamus orders shivering in order to increase the temperature, creating the sensation of severe chills that accompanies the rise in fever. That rise in temperature is so rapid that the victim's teeth chatter and the bed vibrates. Once the new level has been reached, the patient feels terribly hot, and then as the temperature falls, profuse sweating follows, leaving the sufferer washed out and exhausted. In the case of both *vivax* and *falciparum* malaria, this cycle happens at about forty-eight-hour intervals, reflecting the life cycle of the parasite itself. This creates a pattern of fever on day one and then day three, generating the label *tertian* for this cycle. This intermittent pattern helped to distinguish malaria from, say, typhoid fever, which presented with a more continuous fever.

Both *vivax* and *falciparum* can cause chronic illness in circumstances in which the victim endures repeated infection with the parasite. In the chronic case, the spleen remains enlarged, creating a palpable and visible mass in the left side of the abdomen. Since the parasite destroys red blood cells as part of the disease process, the person suffering repeated attacks becomes anemic, weak, and tired. He or she may reach an equilibrium with the parasite, so that active bouts of fever no longer occur, but may never be entirely well. Enervated chronic malaria patients lack the energy for a full workload, be it in school or in the field. During the reduced immune state of pregnancy, malaria may flare, potentially killing the fetus, the mother, or both.

All malaria parasites follow a similar complex life cycle. Part of this occurs within the vertebrate host, and part within the parasite's vector, the anopheles mosquito. The female mosquito takes in the sexual forms of the parasite, called gametocytes, with a blood meal. The gametocytes, male and female, mate in the stomach of the mosquito. The subsequent oocyst burrows into the lining of the mosquito's stomach, undergoes further transformation, and ends up in the mosquito's salivary gland as a long ribbon form called a sporozoite. The mosquito injects the sporozoite into the next person she bites. The parasite's life cycle within the mosquito takes ten to twenty days, depending on climatic conditions. Once injected into the next vertebrate host, the parasite travels first to the liver and then to the red blood cells. It enters a red blood cell, reproduces, and then bursts the red cell to release the newly generated offspring. These may go on to infect other red blood cells, or transform into gametocytes, ready to be taken up by the next biting mosquito. The red-blood-cell-replication phase lasts about forty-eight hours. It is the point of red cell rupture that corresponds with the intermittent fever spikes of malaria.

The life cycle of the parasite is intimately tied to the life cycle of the anopheles mosquito. The female mosquito lays her fertilized eggs in water, where they hatch into larvae. The larval forms then undergo further transformations, finally emerging as the familiar winged insects. The males live off nectar; only the female requires blood meals, for the nourishment of her eggs. The adult mosquito does not fly far from its birthplace, a phenomenon that creates a mosquito zone around wetlands while drier areas may be devoid of mosquito activity. Most anopheles prefer stagnant water for egg laying. Areas near the shoreline that are overgrown with grass or other water plants, clogged with vegetable debris, or protected from wave action make perfect breeding sites. Not only does the stagnant water promote the growth of algae, the principal food source for the larvae, but the debris in the water also blocks access to minnows that might otherwise consume the larvae. While in tropical areas the mosquito breeding cycle continues year round, in the subtropical and temperate climates that characterize most of North America, the mosquito becomes dormant in winter. Egg production stops, so the female is not driven to take blood meals. The mosquitoes hibernate in trees, under houses, and in caves. If the anopheles mosquito is carrying malaria plasmodia when hibernation starts, the organisms usually die over the winter months, although *vivax* malaria has been shown to survive for more than two hundred days in a mosquito host that is warm enough. But most mosquitoes must become newly infected each spring in order to continue transmission.[3]

It is not just the mosquito that is influenced by climatic conditions. Aside from the sharp contrasts of winter and summer, average temperatures are important to the plasmodium as well. For the plasmodium to undergo its one-to-three-week cycle in the mosquito, the ambient air must be warm enough. It matures faster in warmer temperatures, increasing the "turnaround time" and opportunities for new infections. Temperature tolerance differs for the two species of parasite that were most important in the United States. *Falciparum* can complete its development within the mosquito in eight days if the ambient temperature is between 27 and 30 degrees C; reproduction stops below 18 degrees C. *Vivax* can continue development if temperatures drop as low as 9 degrees C, but the appearance of sporozoites (mature infectious forms) takes three weeks. High heat, on the other hand, can stop development as well. Temperatures persistently above 30 degrees C are inimical to parasite development. This threshold determines the patterns of prevalence of these two organisms. *Falciparum* faded out as the latitude rose further from the equator; therefore *falciparum* was a major problem in states south of the thirty-fifth parallel (such as South Carolina and Georgia), and was occasionally seen 100 to 150 miles north of it, but almost never appeared north of the thirty-eighth parallel (say, Cincinnati or so). *Vivax,* on the other hand, at times thrived in southern Canada. In general, it was much more adapted to temperate climates than *falciparum,* which was both more malignant in its effects and more fastidious in its survival requirements.[4]

Climate clearly has a bearing on the density of mosquito breeding and hence the likelihood of malaria transmission. Long hot summers both encourage multiple cycles of mosquito reproduction and speed the development of the parasite within the vector. Throughout the twentieth century malariologists have sought to tie cycles of malaria surges with cyclic changes in the weather. This connection has not turned out to be as clear as might be imagined. Certainly the Mississippi River flood of 1927, whose receding waters created a vast new area for mosquito breeding, brought with it an outbreak of malaria. And the drought years of the early 1930s, which created dust bowls on the plains, accompanied a new low in malaria rates in the South. Closer analyses of malaria mortality rates and rainfall, however, do not show a consistent pattern. For example, when annual rainfall is plotted against malaria mortality for the 1920s, the graphs bear an overall resemblance. But while rainfall stayed about the same from 1922 to 1924, malaria rates dropped sharply, and when rainfall increased markedly in 1926, malaria rates stayed the same.[5] Understanding this conundrum may require paying closer attention to what time of year the rain falls. If the excess rain is concentrated in the first three months, for example, then it will have little effect on mosquito breeding. Also, drought in summer months may actually increase mosquito density, as formerly running streams turn into strings of sluggish puddles, perfect for larval development.

In 1945 Ernest Carroll Faust, a Tulane malariologist who cumulated malaria data for almost three decades, graphed the cycles of malaria mortality over the course of the century. He admitted, "No satisfactory explanation for the cyclic changes in the malaria mortality rate curve has been advanced." He went on to specifically exclude weather cycles. "It does not fit in with solar cycles which have been cited as governing biological trends about every eleven years, and no one has produced a plausible meteorological explanation, although the amount of precipitation may have had some causal connection."[6] An intriguing article appeared late in 1997 that may throw light on this puzzle. Two scientists at the London School of Tropical Medicine and Hygiene looked at the cycles of El Niño and malaria outbreaks in Venezuela during selective periods of the twentieth century. They found that malaria morbidity was increased by an average of 37 percent (P = .004) in the years following recognized El Niño events.[7] It is possible that American malaria cycles are similarly tied to El Niño oscillations, although establishing such a connection is a project for another time.

One characteristic of malaria makes it harder to discern patterns and map them to weather conditions. Malaria parasites may lie dormant in humans for months to years, only to resurface and cause disease even when the person has had no recent contact with malaria-bearing mosquitoes. *Falciparum* malaria displays this behavior to the least degree, relapsing for only a few months after the initial illness and then disappearing. *Vivax*, on the other hand, typically strikes one summer, goes dormant over the winter months, and then recurs in midspring of the following year. Although this can occur again a year later, much longer cycles of relapse are rare. *Malariae* can go on relapsing for years, which can greatly confuse attempts to track malaria and establish whether it is newly occurring in an area. For reasons not at all clear, *vivax* tends to be a disease of the early and midsummer, while *falciparum* strikes in late summer and fall.

## Evolutionary History

Malaria probably afflicted vertebrates before hominids evolved, making us only one of a long series of hosts for this highly successful parasite. The malaria plasmodium may have originated from a free-living plant species, like one of the algae, for it contains fragments of DNA that suggest a lost ability to make chlorophyll. How this algaelike organism made the transition from independent life to a parasitic cycle dependent upon mosquitoes is anyone's guess. Perhaps it started on a stagnant pond where protoplasmodia evolved mechanisms for survival in the larval gut of anopheles mosquitoes. Once it was transformed from the larvae's lunch to its parasite, the jump to vertebrate hosts would have become possible. There are many different malaria plasmodia in nature, specific to birds, lizards, monkeys, apes, cows, and other vertebrates. More than one of the simian malarias can infect humans, although artificial intervention with a syringe is usually required to effect the transfer. Most likely, hominids and malaria evolved side by side, with malaria infecting humans for as long as humans have been in existence.[8]

Of the four malaria parasites that infect humans, which evolved first? And did one evolve from the other? *Falciparum* is the most virulent, and *malariae* the mildest in its effects, while the other two fall in between. One might argue that this implies an older evolutionary age for *malariae,* since humans seem to be more adapted to it. But it turns out that *falciparum* is the closest, in terms of DNA mapping, to simian malarias, making it more likely to resemble the organism that jumped from apes to humans. One resolution to this dilemma is to assume that malaria made the transition from animal to man more than once. Thus *falciparum* could still be the most recently acquired by humans (and hence most virulent), while the others may have plagued humankind longer and come from other more remote sources.[9] The various immunity patterns to malaria offer some clue to this history. Peoples from Africa, the Mediterranean, and South Asia have genetic blood abnormalities that protect them from *falciparum* malaria, not preventing the disease but moderating its course. Most Africans whose genetic heritage goes back to western Africa have total immunity to *vivax* malaria.

This difference in immunity patterns may have helped determine the mildness of *vivax* when compared to *falciparum.* Such a hypothesis lies in the field of disease evolution, which remains a speculative endeavor at best. But recent discussions about the survival value of various levels of virulence spur interesting conjectures. Christopher Wills has argued that one pattern of disease evolution is for a tropical disease to modify its survival requirements in order to expand into temperate environments. The syphilis spirochete, for example, may be the result of a yaws microbe ancestor that found its way out of the tropics. Yaws causes a skin infection and can survive on the skin only in very hot climates. It is very similar in structure to the syphilis parasite. If a yaws spirochete found a way to invade deeper into the human body and come to the surface only in its most "tropical" region (the genitals), then its range would expand outside of the tropics.[10]

Similarly, *vivax* malaria may have evolved from a more virulent tropical ancestor. Back in evolutionary time, when the genetic resistance evolved among some black Africans that rendered them immune to infection, *vivax* faced a crisis. It needed to jump into a new population, but those adjacent, nonimmune populations lived in regions where the anopheles mosquito was dormant during the cold winter months and unavailable for plasmodium transport. Accordingly, the *vivax* organism may have modified its virulence so that its host could live longer, and evolved a mechanism (still poorly understood) by which the coming of spring and the new mosquitoes would be matched by a human malaria relapse, engendering blood rich in parasites. It also evolved to tolerate reproduction within a mosquito that was subjected to colder nighttime temperatures than those common in the tropics.

*Falciparum* faced no such challenges. The existing genetic strategies against malaria infection—sickle-cell trait and G6PD deficiency—did not block infection but rather made it more tolerable by the human host. From the parasite's point of view, this was ideal. The host continued to function and roam, the parasites flourished modestly but sufficiently in the bloodstream, and the chain of infection continued. Paul Ewald has argued that vector-borne diseases have no need to lose virulence, since the prostrate victim becomes even more susceptible to mosquito bites.[11] This may be true in the porous housing conditions of the tropics, but it is less so in the colder north; hence another reason for the lesser virulence of *vivax* compared to *falciparum.* In any event, *falciparum* retains its virulence in Africa to this day, and it certainly had a major impact on the subtropical areas of the New World. *Vivax,* on the other hand, has largely died out in the temperate regions of North America and Europe.

## Malaria, Race, and Immunity

The complexities of malaria immunity reflect humankind's long struggle with this parasite and are inextricably interwoven with a particular individual's race, place of origin, and time spent in malarious areas in recent years. Any person who survives in a hyperendemic malarious area will eventually come into some sort of equilibrium with the local malaria parasites, which implies that the immune system has gained some power over the invading organism. This is not absolute; as the difficulties in manufacturing a malaria vaccine illustrate, simple complete immunity against malarial parasites cannot be acquired through exposure. But acquired partial immunity, after a time of "seasoning" in the malarious area, will allow a person to function and work, even though not necessarily at full strength or health.

Genetic immunities, or protective inborn traits that are directly determined by an individual's DNA, are much more complex and varied than the acquired immunity that any person can achieve if occupying a malarious area long enough. Discussing genetic immunities takes us into the domain of racial medicine, for the presence of these traits tends to sort by race, making them potential biological markers of the human subspecies, a highly controversial topic. Malaria, more than any other disease, forces the question: is race a purely social construct or a significant biological reality? Modern anthropologists argue that races do not exist, for the human species cannot be divided in any meaningful way by such superficial characteristics as skin color, facial traits, and hair texture. From a genetic point of view, one racial group cannot be distinguished from another; there is great variety in the human phenotype, but those differences blend and meld, rather than standing in distinct clusters. On this view, race cannot be defined biologically. This is particularly evident in the varying definitions of race across culture. Americans tend to think in terms of the "one-drop rule"; having only one black ancestor defines a person as black. Other cultures have distinct categories for brown- versus-black-skinned people, or they distinguish Asian races by country of origin. Obviously, race is a social creation, one that has often served to oppress and control large groups of people during European expansion and imperialism.[12]

Arguments against the existence of races are compelling. If they stir opposition, it is likely to be formulated in terms of differences in malaria resistance and the sickle-cell hemoglobin trait among "races." According to this point of view, it is reasonable to use the marker of black skin as a determinant of a certain epidemiological category. People who are black are both more likely to have abnormal hemoglobin and are more likely to be resistant to malaria. Hence the concept of the black race has a nontrivial biological reality, one that makes a difference in disease prevalence. This line of reasoning can be expanded into the social realm as well. Because Africans are less susceptible to malaria, they were able to survive and reproduce in tropical and subtropical environments where malaria was endemic. This included the warmest regions of the New World, which from the sixteenth century onward were ripe for agricultural exploitation by Europeans. The European master's claim that only blacks were suited to work on Caribbean, Brazilian, or South Carolinian plantations had some truth. Race is an important and real biological category; it has implications for epidemiology, and epidemiology has had profound historical consequences.

The example of malaria can be extended to other diseases, although not with such clarity. There is more hypertension among American blacks than whites, for example, and tuberculosis is more prevalent among them.[13] Black mothers have smaller babies on average than whites, and blacks may be more susceptible to frostbite. Articles published in major medical journals such as the *New England Journal of Medicine* have explored these differences with the clear underlying assumption that race is a definable biological variable, comparable to age or sex.[14] Yet in 1984 the use of race as an epidemiological category was thoroughly condemned by a medical author who rightly pointed out that there is no way, other than self-labeling, to say what race any person belongs to.[15] Authors struggle to be moral on this issue as well as right. It can be argued that race is mainly a proxy for class, and hence studies that find a correlation between tuberculosis and race, for example, are really about a correlation between tuberculosis and poverty and oppression, not skin color.[16] Only right-wing racists, this line of argument sometimes continues, would blame tuberculosis on color (an unchangeable variable) rather than socioeconomic conditions, which are amenable to intervention.

This discussion becomes even more complex because of the particular difficulties of studying blacks and disease. The Tuskegee syphilis study tops anyone's list of abuses that have been administered in the name of American medical research. Clearly that study, with its lack of informed consent and denial of curative treatment, was immoral and racist.[17] But does that mean any study that uses race as a variable is invariably racist? On the contrary, some civil rights activists say that the medical establishment has ignored blacks (and women), testing drugs primarily on white males. Since the drugs then used by doctors may be inappropriate for blacks and women, these patients are oppressed by the racist/sexist researchers who refuse to study blacks and women. These groups have a *right* to have drugs tested on them, these activists argue, so that their medical care can be tailored to their needs. Julius Chambers, chancellor emeritus of historically black North Carolina Central University (NCCU) and prominent civil rights spokesman, made this attitude the centerpiece of his plans for the university's growth in the new millenium. He wanted NCCU to become a leader in the pathophysiological study of black Americans, because their medical needs had been too long ignored.[18] The same inspiration underlies research on African-Americans and hypertension at Wake Forest School of Medicine, and the publication of a textbook entirely on black health issues.[19]

Epidemiologists are thus caught in a moral dilemma: how to handle race appropriately as a research variable, giving it proper attention, while at the same time balancing biological determinism with sensitivity to socioeconomic forces. They experience political pressure to come up with the "right" answer, the answer that further establishes the burden of oppression and poverty that has been the African-American's experience. Thus the differential in tuberculosis morbidity rates "should" be due to poverty, and queries about local immune function in the lungs of blacks are inherently suspicious. Likewise, the lower birth weights of black infants "should" be a marker of socioeconomic plight and not due to some inherited intrinsic factor. Researchers have been sensitive to these concerns, and recent articles on tuberculosis and infant birth weight have striven to control for socioeconomic status, so that influence of race per se can be assessed. In both these instances, blacks are at a disadvantage, but those vigilant against biological determinism want at all costs to avoid any insinuation that blacks are somehow inferior beings. This vigilance is most necessary, as might be expected, when the intelligence and college performance of black and white students are compared. There can be no doubt that the "right" answer is that the economic disadvantage of blacks determines their lower test scores; any discussion of biological determinism in this setting immediately brings on accusations of racism.[20]

But what of malaria? Here is a circumstance in which Africans and their descendants are stronger than other groups, more able to fight a disease and survive environmental stresses. Even this strength has served the forces of oppression, though, since it was used to justify slavery. Those fearful of the oppressive powers of biological determinism shy away from fully acknowledging the implications of this hereditary difference. They tend instead to focus on acquired immunities rather than inherited ones, for these are dependent only on place of residence, not on color of skin. This book argues that the biological and social parameters of malaria and race need to be faced head on. In the history of malaria in the United States, race does matter, but so does socioeconomic status, with its determinacy of the quality and location of housing, access to medical care, and level of nutrition. The links between malaria and race are accidents of environmental history; it just so happened that malaria and black-skinned Africans overlapped in space and time for enough generations that inherited immunities evolved. One might expand this observation to speculate that the disease burden of sub-Saharan Africa helped create a situation in which the population was vulnerable to capture and enslavement, but that is a topic for another day. In any event, the fact remains that black men and women who were brought unwillingly to the New World carried in their genes some protection against malaria.

Discussions about the relationship of malaria and race are dominated by questions about modes of immunity. The spectrum of protective bodily responses to malaria is one of the most intricate systems of immune response known for any infectious disease. It reflects millennia of interaction and evolution and is a historical phenomenon of both the population from which the individual emerges as well as that individual's personal life experiences. It is not surprising that such complexities were not fully explicated until the mid-twentieth century; it is also not surprising that some variation in the susceptibility of black and white to malaria was noted early on in the mutual interaction of the two races in the tropics.

One way to tease apart this web of defenses against malaria is to follow the life events of one person. Let's look at a girl in Africa, who is born and raised in a highly malarious area, Kenya. At birth she already has two kinds of inheritance that will protect her from malaria in the first months and years of her life. This advantage is necessary for her survival, since the mosquitoes begin biting her at once, injecting her with malaria parasites. Like all infants, she carries immune substances acquired from her mother's blood during pregnancy. She also maintains access to her mother's immune system through breast-feeding. Thus she shares, for a short period of time, in her mother's acquired immunity to malaria (discussed in more detail below). She may also have a genetic heritage that protects her— abnormalities in her red blood cells that make it more difficult for the malaria parasite to become established in her body.[21]

The best known of these abnormalities is hemoglobin S, the underlying abnormality in sickle-cell anemia. In this disorder a single mutation in the gene coding for hemoglobin production leads to a functional but malformed hemoglobin molecule. Hemoglobin is the substance inside the red blood cell that carries oxygen, so it is crucial to life. The Kenyan girl inherits genes for hemoglobin production from both of her parents. If she gets the gene for hemoglobin S, the sickle-cell gene, from both parents, she will have sickle-cell anemia, a disease that leads to early death unless modern medical care is available. But if she gets one normal hemoglobin gene and one abnormal one, she will be healthy and is said to have sickle-cell trait (but not disease). For reasons still not clear to medical science, having sickle-cell trait gives her some resistance to *falciparum* malaria. This is not an absolute immunity, but rather a factor that increases her chance of surviving the first years of life. It continues to help into adulthood, although its importance diminishes.

Other genetic "defects" also help the infant girl survive malaria. The immature form of hemoglobin that all fetuses make (fetal hemoglobin or hemoglobin F) makes red blood cells less receptive to the malaria parasite and offers protection for as long as it lasts (the early months of life). Some children appear to produce hemoglobin F longer than others, a genetic "defect" that can protect them against illness. Less common than sickle-cell hemoglobin but present in West Africa is another type of abnormal hemoglobin, hemoglobin C. Like hemoglobin S, the hemoglobin C gene, if received from both parents, causes anemia and shortens life, but if the child has half normal, half hemoglobin C, she has adequate oxygen-carrying capacity as well as a shield against malaria. A similar situation exists for the inherited metabolic disorder G6PD deficiency. It may also be true of another form of inherited anemia, thallasemia, which is found in peoples who historically have lived in the malarious regions of India, Southwest Asia, and the Mediterranean. Malaria's tendency to kill young children makes it a powerful evolutionary force, capable of selecting for and maintaining anything that gives a child an advantage in the struggle for life.

There is one form of malaria parasite that the Kenyan child will probably not acquire at all: *Plasmodium vivax*. About 95 percent of sub-Saharan Africans have a characteristic of their red blood cells that causes them no apparent harm—the absence of a cell-wall structure called the Duffy antigen. Without this antigen, the *vivax* parasite apparently cannot gain entrance into the red blood cell. This represents an absolute immunity; bearers of "Duffy-negative" red blood cells will never have *vivax* malaria, although under certain circumstances the parasites may be swimming in their bloodstreams. They can, in other words, be infected but not sick at all.[22]

The situation for *falciparum* malaria is very different. Most adults living in a highly malarious area will have *falciparum* parasites in their blood, and while not acutely ill, they will not be fully well either. By definition they have survived childhood, due to having sufficient food, clothing, and parental care; they may have benefited as well from maternal antibodies, hemoglobin variants, or other genetic characteristics. *Falciparum* parasites have been likely omnipresent in their bloodstreams all the days of their lives. With that prolonged exposure comes a partial tolerance, so-called acquired immunity, which marks the infected but functioning individual. But maintenance of the full degree of tolerance requires continual exposure. When such adults are taken out of the malarious area, they will gradually lose their resistance to *falciparum* (although never entirely). This acquired malaria tolerance does not depend on the presence of hemoglobin S but is a tautologous sort of phenomenon—if a person survives for a given period of time in an area infested with *falciparum* malaria, then he is a survivor, a person who has acquired tolerance. Black Africans may have a "leg up" on this survival because of hemoglobin variants or other traits that help them survive childhood, but anyone who can survive can become tolerant and hence benefit from acquired immunity.

So let us return to our Kenyan girl mentioned above. Suppose she survives the many challenges of early childhood to become a woman. She carries *falciparum* in her blood and is probably less robust and less energetic than she might have been without it, but she is generally in moderately good health. During pregnancy she may well have attacks of malaria, for the immune function is in general damped during pregnancy in order to tolerate the foreign matter of the fetus. Malaria may indeed kill her or kill the baby in utero. But if she and the infant survive, the cycle of protection and tolerance will begin again. The disease thus lives in balance with her people, for the healthy adults serve as able carriers, perpetuating the disease in the population while at the same time tolerating it within their own bodies.

The scenario sketched here is most applicable to a stable African village and is of varying applicability in the Americas. Certainly many adults who were forcibly removed from Africa to the New World carried *falciparum* parasites within their tolerant bodies, allowing the chain of infection to leap to the American colonies. But in some instances the infection would have died out, causing the African-Americans to lose the acquired component of their immunity. Any ethnic population raised with a variable exposure to malaria would have had the same experience. A child—white, black, or Asian—who grew up in a highly malarious area would have acquired partial immunity as an adult. If he or she then moved away to a place without malaria, that protection would fade, so that over time a community highly susceptible to epidemic malaria might evolve. Race might well help predict childhood survival from malaria, but in adults acquired immunities are probably more important for understanding the pattern of malaria acquisition and morbidity.

## Malaria in the Americas

This discussion of the biology, genetics, and epidemiology of malaria forms the backdrop for understanding the course of malaria in the Americas. Biology is central to determining whether malaria was indigenous to the New World or was imported by Europeans or Asians. The earliest humans came to the American continents over a land bridge that crossed the Bering Strait from present-day Russia into Alaska. Those peoples walked down through the plains of Canada into North, Central, and South America. Any diseases they endured had to either travel with their bodies or be already present in the hemisphere when they arrived. It is likely that they found mosquitoes in abundance—but were they loaded with malarial parasites? Did these peoples bring any parasites with them?

The answer to both questions is almost certainly no. Active cases of malaria are unlikely to have survived passage through the "cold screen" of northern Asia and Alaska. Doing so would have required continuous transmission to anopheles mosquitoes, reinfection of new hosts, and persistence of the disease through generations. Given how much time must have passed before these people again reached lands with a climate hospitable to malaria, the parasite could not have survived. A second possibility is that malaria evolved from simian to human separately in the New World, so that transmission was not dependent upon passage across the Bering Strait. But this too is unlikely, because only a small number of monkey species carry plasmodia in the Americas, whereas they are found throughout the primate and mammalian world of Asia and Africa. Rather, malaria was most likely introduced late into the Western Hemisphere from outside. The strongest argument for this conclusion is the lack of genetic protection against the disease among Native Americans. Whereas sickle-cell trait, thallasemia, and other hemoglobinopathies map intimately with malarious areas elsewhere in the world, no such protective factors appear in Native Americans. One anthropologist has even argued that the near 100 percent frequency of the O blood type among Native Americans is another indication that malaria has been introduced only recently to these peoples. The AB blood type, she argues, which is not as advantageous in other ways as O, offers some protection against mosquito bites. A person with the AB blood type would thus be at lower risk for acquiring malaria (although at higher risk for other health problems). Where malaria has prevailed, the AB blood type should prevail likewise. Where malaria has been unknown for hundreds of generations, the AB blood type should be rare, which is the case among the indigenous peoples of America. In any event, malaria has left no discernible biological footprints to suggest that it has existed among Native Americans long enough for them to evolve inborn characteristics against the disease.[23]

Localized outbreaks may have occured in the centuries before Columbus, without the disease necessarily being indigenous to the Americas. Malaria could have arrived in boats bearing Vikings or Arabs or Japanese or other Asians anytime after 900 C.E. or so, when such ships could have survived an ocean crossing.[24] Scattered pre-Columbian outbreaks aside, Europeans undoubtedly brought malaria to the New World in the decades after 1492. Did malaria play a role in what David Stannard has called the "American Holocaust," the wholesale devastation of Native Americans by European diseases (as well as European guns)?[25] It is possible but hard to determine with certainty. Most commonly, smallpox is cited as the disease that most ravaged the native population, and measles a close second. In trying to make such retrospective diagnoses, however, we must rely on sixteenth- and seventeenth-century observers, a procedure fraught with many sources of error. These men may have been seeing something never previously documented by Europeans—the effect of microbes on a virgin population with no acquired or genetic immunity to them. The microbes may have been predominantly the smallpox and measles viruses, but some other organism in the common oral flora of Europeans, completely innocuous to its original host, may also have caused these native epidemics. Whether malaria was part of this mass killing is very hard to know, although later, when African workers arrived, there is commentary that Native Americans could not live in the same areas with the Africans, because the Americans died so rapidly with fevers.[26]

This question of Native American susceptibility can be approached another way. Are there recorded episodes of new contact between malaria carriers and Native Americans that happened more recently and hence are more available for study? An intriguing disease outbreak during the early 1830s may meet this description. Beginning in 1829 and lasting through 1834, an epidemic raged on the western coast of North America, from the Sacramento River valley of central California northward into Vancouver and British Columbia. The best account of this outbreak comes from physicians and other literate men stationed at Fort Vancouver, a trading post in the Oregon territory. They reported a fearsome occurrence of fever with a high native mortality. Almost all of the Caucasians became ill, but deaths were few among them. The Indians, however, died in droves. One clergyman wrote about his trip to Oregon in 1835, "I have found the Indian population . . . below the falls of the Columbia, far less than I had expected, or what it was when Lewis and Clarke [*sic*] made their tour. Since the year 1829, probably seven-eighths, if not as Dr. McLoughlin believes, nine-tenths, have been swept away by the disease." He called the outbreak "fever and ague" and claimed that villages and even whole tribes had just disappeared. The natives died so fast that heaps of unburied dead could be seen from the riverbank. Another observer in the Sacramento River valley commented in 1834, "Many of the native Indians have perished. . . . Many tribes are utterly extinct; in places where I was told that, in 1832, there was a population of a thousand or fifteen hundred souls, I found sometimes but one hundred." There, too, piles of human bones bespoke a rapid plague that left no one to bury the dead.[27]

Was this outbreak malaria? It struck in July, raged until midfall, and then disappeared, only to reoccur in the same season a year later. If the epidemic was influenza—perhaps the leading alternative candidate—the seasonality makes no sense. The few contemporary accounts all agree in using terms usually associated with malaria—fever and ague, intermittent fever, tertian fever. Otherwise the description of the malady is fairly non-specific—high fevers and diffuse pains. No rash is mentioned, which rules out smallpox. Malaria could easily have been imported from the eastern United States or Spanish dominions south of California. The Euro-Americans at Fort Vancouver improved with quinine, whereas the Native Americans had no access to this drug. Still, the appalling mortality is unlike that of malaria, especially *vivax* malaria, which would almost certainly be the organism in question, given the geography and yearly relapse pattern. Perhaps this is what malaria looks like in a truly virgin population, with no acquired or inherited immunities at all, to either *vivax* or *falciparum.*

If malaria affected Native Americans this way, the pattern shows up only rarely elsewhere. I have only found one other reference to severe Native American mortality from what may have been malaria. One Thomas Nuttall, traveling in Arkansas territory in 1819, reported, "From July to October the ague and bilious fever spread throughout the territory in a very unusual manner. . . . The paroxysms attended with excruciating pain, took place every other day, similar to the common intermittent." What was unusual about the epidemic was the significant mortality among the native inhabitants. "I was credibly informed," he continued, "that not less than one hundred of the Cherokees, settled contiguous to the banks of the Arkansas died this season of the bilious fever."[28] Other tribes did have trouble with malaria, especially when forced into resettlement by the U.S. authorities. Arapaho and Cheyenne tribes were afflicted by malaria in the

1880s, for example, when they were relocated west of the Missouri River. But their mortality was apparently not as excessive as appears to have been the case half a century earlier. Perhaps they were not as "virgin" then, having been through prior outbreaks? It is hard to know whether the Oregon territory events were typical but generally not observed by white reporters, or wildly atypical. Still, it does appear that malaria should be included among the European diseases that helped clear the way for Caucasian conquest of North America.[29]

Two different malarial parasites came to the New World, one from Europe and one from Africa. They have separate histories. Europeans brought *vivax* malaria; Africans brought *falciparum*. *Vivax* malaria was common in England, Holland, Spain, and Italy, all countries that supplied explorers and settlers to North America from the earliest days of European invasion. While these Europeans carried the *vivax* parasites in their bodies, they also had genetic and acquired immunities to malaria. To be sure, they were not invulnerable to infection, nor equally immune. But these European settlers were unlikely to experience the "virgin soil effect" upon exposure to *vivax*—that is, high mortality rates. Africans carried little *vivax*, since they had acquired almost total immunity to this infection. Rather, they transported *falciparum* parasites and with them various degrees of immunity to infection. Again, their immunity was not total for adults and was even weaker for children. Still, Africans in the New World would have had no risk of disease from *vivax* and lower morbidity and mortality from *falciparum* than Europeans. Most European settlers, for their part, would have had no "genetic memory" of *falciparum* and, at least initially, no acquired immunity. Predictably, when Europeans and Africans met in the subtropical and tropical climates of America, a high morbidity and mortality rate from *falciparum* malaria among the Europeans was the inevitable result.[30]

The date when malaria arrived in the North American colonies is disputed, but *vivax* was probably established in the middle and northern colonies by 1700. In a pattern that would be repeated again and again as European settlement progressed across the continent, the colonists first settled close to their main form of transportation and source of power: water. Both bays and rivers had still water, suitable for mosquito breeding. As grain production increased and mills were needed, streams were dammed for water power. The resultant mill ponds added to the opportunities for mosquito larvae. The earliest housing was porous, further increasing mosquito exposure. From Penobscot Bay to the James River, *vivax* malaria flourished, albeit with greater and greater vivacity the more southern the colony. Given the low population density throughout colonial North America, *vivax* appeared in some places (such as the Chesapeake) as a chronic disease and elsewhere as epidemic outbreaks separated by relatively disease-free years. It waxed and waned in severity, perhaps because different strains of *vivax* were prevalent, with populations having acquired immunity to one but not another.[31]

*Vivax* was introduced many times into the North American colonies, but when the first outbreak occurred is unclear. One candidate for the first epidemic among Englishmen was the devastating fever that raged at Jamestown in the early years of its settlement. English adventurers first settled Jamestown in 1607. Over the next decade more than seventeen hundred immigrants arrived, but two-thirds of them did not survive more than a year or two. Many problems plagued the settlers, including malnutrition and Native American attacks. But a major source of mortality was a deadly fever that affected almost every colonist.

Some historians believe this fever was malaria, in part because Jamestown is located on a peninsula surrounded by swamps. Early accounts speak of agues, fevers, chills, and fluxes. Fevers and chills are nonspecific symptoms of many infectious diseases, while fluxes are diarrheal illnesses. The word *ague* came to be used fairly exclusively for malaria during the nineteenth century, but this usage was not so specific in the early seventeenth century. The Jamestown settlers came from England, including parts of England where *vivax* malaria was common. They certainly could have brought it with them. But one would not expect such a nonvirgin population, however malnourished, to experience a major outbreak of *vivax* malaria with that level of mortality. Could the disease have been *falciparum* malaria? Again, it is unlikely: Africans did not arrive in Jamestown before 1619, and there was no other obvious source of the *falciparum* parasite. Most likely, as historians Wyndham Blanton and Carville Earle have argued, the malignant disease suffered in Jamestown was typhoid fever, spread through the unsanitary habits of the colonists, who lived cheek by jowl in a tiny fort. Earle argues in addition that the Jamestown water supply would frequently have been high in salt, leading to edema and serious health consequences.[32]

The arrival of *falciparum* malaria in North America is easier to pinpoint, since its impact on European colonists was so dire. It first appeared in South Carolina during the 1680s, where the climate was warm enough for *falciparum* to flourish, and the mosquitoes breeding in the coastal lowlands swarmed over the settlers. The rich land rewarded the cultivation of rice and indigo, which could be easily transported by river and coastal waters to the port of Charleston. According to historian Peter Wood, the area was relatively healthy until the 1680s, when a new form of infectious disease began to raise mortality rates. Not coincidentally, the importation of black slaves accelerated in the 1680s, and *falciparum* was probably imported then as well. The mortality among white settlers was high, approaching Caribbean levels. Africans appeared to find the climate less deadly, which reinforced their use as slaves. Hence more Africans were brought in, and more malaria, continuing the deadly cycle. *Vivax* was probably present too, in the European immigrants, but it did not begin to make the mortality dent that *falciparum* did.[33]

*Falciparum* malaria had a major impact on South Carolina's history. Historian Peter Coclanis has noted that the colony did not begin to sustain itself naturally (that is, by births rather than incoming immigrants) until the 1770s, a century after it was settled. By studying low country parish registers, he found data "at once more ghastly and more incredible." One register showed that 86 percent of white babies born died before they reached age 20; in another, 2,883 burials were recorded against 863 baptisms (all white persons). While this excessive mortality was not all due to *falciparum,* it played a major role.[34] As would happen elsewhere when malaria moved into a landscape, South Carolina's settlers bemoaned the "paradise lost" that had once been their home. The area had been salubrious on first settlement, with only a few light fevers, nothing troublesome. But by the early years of the eighteenth century, the colony had acquired a reputation for unwholesomeness. An English proverb of the time ran "They who want to die quickly, go to Carolina," a sentiment echoed by a German observer who wrote, "Carolina is in the spring a paradise, in the summer a hell and in the autumn a hospital."[35]

Reports of high mortality had a dramatic effect on the settlement of South Carolina. The relative African immunity to malaria and yellow fever created optimal circumstances for the expansion of African slavery and the near absence of indentured or free white immigrant labor. Immigration to Carolina slowed markedly, and the whites that did live there made adjustments in an attempt to limit the disease. Those wealthy enough traveled elsewhere during the malarious months, escaping the swampy lowlands for the pine hills, mountains, seacoast, or northern states. Charleston was actually relatively healthy, since the mosquitoes that bred in its salty marshes were not effective malaria carriers, a factor that contributed to town growth. By the time of the Revolution and beyond, the colony had a black majority, a situation that would fuel strong attitudes toward slavery and its control in the nineteenth century, when sectional differences threatened the peculiar institution.[36]

Malaria was also a major health problem in the colonial Chesapeake, as historians Darrett and Anita Rutman have documented. They have studied the differential mortality experiences of the Virginia and Maryland colonies compared with those of New England. While agreeing that the presence of malaria in seventeenth-century Virginia was controversial, the Rutmans join other historians in concluding that the disease was rampant in the eighteenth century, and that it had a major impact on mortality. They further suggest that this mortality had broad-ranging implications, affecting patterns of land holding, family structure, and cultural life. It certainly affected the colonies' prosperity and limited demographic growth.[37]

Malaria appeared farther north, in New York, Pennsylvania, and New England, but it was less of a burden. The best account of the New England experience comes from Oliver Wendell Holmes of Massachusetts, who surveyed local physicians in the 1830s for their memories of malaria in earlier years, in addition to culling information from written sources. Holmes shared the assumption, common to his time, that marshes, swamps, and lakes caused malarial fevers, but he was at a loss to explain why the disease had largely died out in New England. Judging from his account, most malaria in recent memory had occurred around mill ponds, and indeed Holmes labeled such ponds a "focus of malaria." He used a map to chronicle cases around one particular pond to emphasize the geographical correlation. Although he did not go beyond the miasmatic theory of intermittent fever's etiology, his map conclusively demonstrates that something about the pond generated this particular fever. Holmes was also interested in a legal case in Lichtfield, Connecticut, tried in January 1800. Some of the townspeople, tired of experiencing recurrent fevers in the neighborhood of one such pond, tore down the dam that sustained it. The dam's owner sued for damages, and the defendants countered that the dam was a public nuisance and its destruction justified. The judge eventually found for the plaintiff, but only after extensive expert testimony that stagnant water generated malarial fevers.[38]

Tracking malaria in the American colonies is complicated by the disease's varying etymology. If one illness label used in the colonial era corresponds to the modern notion of malaria, it is *ague*. But this was not a time of precise diagnosis, or even of the assumption that discrete disease categories existed. Some English physicians, such as Thomas Sydenham, did try to distinguish one fever from another and wrote classic descriptions of rheumatic fever and tuberculosis. Most medical and lay writers of the sixteenth through eighteenth centuries, however, thought in terms of fevers in general, whose symptoms were modified by local environment, season, gender, climate, previous susceptibility, and perhaps even astrological influences. The phrase "fever and ague" recurs frequently in colonial discussions of disease. Many of these episodes probably were caused by plasmodia, but the term *ague* could mean chills or shaking in general as well. Thus, just as modern physicians speak of "chills and fever" as a single symptomatic unit, "fever and ague" could have been used to describe any febrile event. How a particular writer applied the phrase needs to be determined from other evidence, such as the association with swampy ground, the appearance of the disease in the summer months, and the display of the "tawny tone" or skin color that suggests jaundice. Twentieth-century physicians had trouble diagnosing malaria with certainty into the 1940s, so retrospective diagnosis to the colonial era should be made with both care and humility.[39]

Colonial Americans were not powerless against these ravaging epidemics. They had two weapons with which to fight: cinchona bark and relocation. Cinchona (or chinchona) bark from the Peruvian cinchona tree was introduced into Spain in 1640, where it was also known as Peruvian bark, Jesuit's bark, or just the bark. Hailed as a general remedy against fevers, it spurred hot debate among seventeenth-century medical professionals, especially in England. The bark, which includes among other active ingredients quinine, has a mild antipyretic effect and a far stronger impact in cases of malaria. The bark was so popular that it no doubt opened a market for fraudulent imitations and adulterated mixtures, but it was at least available. So while a simplistic statement that colonials "had quinine and knew it was good for malaria" would be far from accurate, colonial physicians did have knowledge of, and access to, a drug that could quell malarial fevers.[40]

Perhaps the more important weapon against malaria was relocation to a more healthful environment. Since the time of ancient Greek medicine, when Hippocrates wrote *Airs, Waters, and Places,* the association had been made between hot, swampy areas and bad health. Lowlands were prone to be sickly, while highlands were healthy. The hot and humid summer and early fall seasons were dangerous times to be in the lowlands, and relocation at such times promoted health. This knowledge suggested strategies to colonial Americans that empirically proved successful. Living away from swampy land or flooded rice fields, preferably on the highest point of land around, offered protection from the summer fevers. Leaving lowlands altogether for higher ground had a similar effect. Draining of swampy areas improved the health of those in proximity, and locating towns away from swamps diminished morbidity. All of these lessons were learned through harsh experience, and they were explained in terms of poisonous airs or miasms; not until the late nineteenth century was it understood that the cause of disease was not a swamp's noxious vapors but its pesky mosquitoes.

Colonists thus labeled certain colonies as healthy and others as dangerous. The correlation with latitude was not missed by immigrants in choosing where to settle. The Caribbean was understood to be the most dangerous, with Florida and Carolina being a close second. The Chesapeake was a bit healthier, but only in New York, New England, and Pennsylvania did the European colonists thrive, produce large families, and prosper as farmers.[41] Much has been made of the relationship between malaria tolerance and the choice of Africans as the laborers of the subtropical colonies. Certainly, as Philip Curtin has argued, the ability of black adults to function in a highly malarious environment made them more valuable as workers, especially in the Caribbean, where the disease pressure brought by malaria was much higher than in the Carolina lowlands.[42] By the turn of the eighteenth century, when malaria was likely entrenched in the Chesapeake and Carolina low country, the reputation of these regions as healthful and attractive had plummeted, generating demand for involuntary African laborers. While no simple cause and effect can be directly established, and other diseases such as yellow fever certainly played their part, it can at least be concluded that malaria had a substantial impact on labor and settlement patterns in the American colonies, patterns that would ultimately lead to the Civil War.

Toward the end of the eighteenth century, medical parlance moved toward greater exactitude, as the profession understood fevers with greater specificity. Although the label *intermittent fever* had been used at least as early as 1609, in the eighteenth and nineteenth centuries it came to characterize the disease now called malaria. As with the term *ague,* the mapping was not exact. Many viral illnesses, as well as tuberculosis and some malignancies, may feature waxing and waning fevers, and these would have offered confusion. "Intermitting" fevers were often contrasted to "continued" ones, which included typhoid and typhus. Other adjectives might be applied, such as *putrid, malignant,* or *remittent,* in order to bring greater precision and prognostic skill to the bedside assessment. Further, the classic case of intermittent fever, with the smooth pattern of forty-eight-hour cycles, usually occurred only in the malaria "virgin" who was entering a malarious country for the first time. Seasoned residents would have bouts of illness, spiking chills and fever, and other manifestations, but since they combined steady exposure to the parasite with some degree of acquired immunity, they rarely displayed the clear pattern that textbooks described. Hence true intermittents were seasoning illnesses; locals never got them— because they already had them. Still, the use of the term *intermittent* began to distinguish medical language from that of the common folk, who continued to complain of agues. The transition was never absolute, but the trend is evident both in nineteenth-century medical writing and in the many frontier lay works that refer to agues.

Malaria was certainlly present among Revolutionary War soldiers. While Wyndham Blanton may well be right that it was not an important disease in seventeenth-century Virginia, during the Revolutionary War it hovered over the James River peninsula and raided both armies as the southern campaign drew to its close. The area around Yorktown is boggy and buggy and no doubt bred abundant mosquitoes that plagued the troops of Washington and Cornwallis alike. While both remittents and intermittents simultaneously prevailed—most likely, a mixture of malaria and typhoid—fully a third of the patients at an American field hospital near Yorktown in 1781 were listed as suffering from intermittent fever. Similar casualties affected

Nathaniel Greene's troops camped outside of Charleston in 1782; half of his men were incapacitated by fevers, and malaria predominated in the disease lists, again with its companion typhoid.[43]

Here and always, malaria was more of an enervating disease than one that caused high mortality. The man suffering from fever and chills often did not die (especially if the disease was *vivax*), but he could no more take part in a battle than he could follow a plow. Malaria generated weakness, lassitude, and a lack of industry that could be especially limiting in the military or frontier setting. Cinchona compounds helped get men back on their feet and were an important factor in the Revolutionary War as well as in the settlement of the early American frontier. While the active ingredient, quinine, rarely cures *vivax* malaria, it does suppress the disease, allowing men and women to plant crops, build houses, dig drainage ditches, and tend livestock—all activities that would lead to increased resistance to malaria, and to prosperity in general.[44]

By 1800 malaria was fading in the Northeast, persisting in the South, and expanding along the frontier. Physicians and laypersons alike knew that intermittent fever was the result of bad air, especially the air arising from foul, stagnant water. They had cinchona bark to help subdue the shaking fits that made life hell for the unfortunate every three days. The visage of the malaria sufferer was a familiar feature of warm climates and the frontier—sallow, weak, haggard. The face was so common among southern and pioneer farmers that it was just part of the expected scene. For another hundred years malaria would dominate the rural experience of America's rougher areas, until social and scientific changes would force it to retreat and hide out in the American South until well into the twentieth century.

As the nineteenth century opened, malignant mists were thought to cause malarial fevers; one hundred years later a complex chain of parasite and mosquito explained the disease. Over the course of the century, malaria afflicted the American frontier, helping produce the roughness and hardship that defined frontier life in contrast to more eastern civilization. During at least some decades of the nineteenth century, malaria affected all regions significantly and severely damaged the health of troops in the Civil War. Toward the end of the century, however, the disease retreated, so that by 1900 it was largely a disease of the southern states. What had been a disease of all parts of the United States became in the twentieth century one more indicator of the poverty, backwardness, and unhealthiness of the South.

## Malaria on the Frontier

While malaria declined in the northeastern states, it grew briskly along the westward-moving line of the frontier. When the lands across the Appalachians became available for settlement, Euro-Americans flowed through gaps and down rivers that took them into Ohio, Indiana, Illinois, Kentucky, Tennessee, and states farther south. As families traveled for days by flatboat and set up flimsy camps near the water, their transportation connection to goods and markets, malaria blossomed. During the antebellum period the wave of malaria subsided in these initial encampments as sturdier houses were built farther off the water, while at the same time it moved on to even newer camps farther west and north. Malaria, most of it *vivax,* became a common feature of raw frontier life, defining in part what it meant to be in the woods, beyond civilization, beyond the safe life of "back home."[1]

Malaria had traditionally been viewed, at least in the more temperate climates of Europe, as a country disease. David Ramsay, a South Carolina physician writing in the late eighteenth century, typically noted that intermittent fevers first appeared after an area had been cleared to make way for settlements and farms. So there was an initial stage without disease, followed by chronic ill health from marsh fevers. But as cities such as Charleston grew, the land became progressively better drained and the location healthier. "It has long been observed in the low countries," Ramsay wrote, "that they who reside in towns, are more healthy than they who live dispersed in the country."[2] Given its association with swamps, malaria declined where people built clusters of houses. It was general knowledge that low, wet lands made bad sites for dwellings or towns; such areas were prone to both flooding and disease. So towns tended to be built on the higher elevations in a region, where the topography encouraged drainage. This tendency was countered by the need for populations to cluster near modes of transportation, and before the advent of railroads in the 1840s, that meant near bodies of water. Some cities, such as Charleston, were favored by sandy soil that drained easily and by surrounding salt marshes that were inhospitable to disease-carrying anophelines. Other cities, just by dint of construction, paving, and drainage, broke the malaria chain by denying anophelines the requisite swampy expanse within a mile of human populations. Hence even in the relatively rural American South and early frontier, as towns became established, malaria withdrew to the countryside.

This was evident to medical observers in the South, who sometimes contrasted the preferences of malaria and yellow fever for different stages of settlement. Mobile physician Josiah Clark Nott commented in 1847, for example: "When the forest is first leveled and a town commenced, intermittents and remittents spring up." So malaria was tied to breaking new ground on the frontier. Yellow fever, however, came later: "As the population increases, the town spreads, and draining and paving are introduced," he continued, "yellow fever, the mighty monarch of the South, who scorns the rude field and forest, plants his sceptre in the centre, and drives all other fevers to the outskirts."[3] This would become a recurring theme throughout malaria's course in the United States. It was associated with rough, frontier conditions, not with the increasing civilization of towns and cities.

Perhaps the best description of this phenomenon comes to us from the pen of Charles Dickens, who traveled the Ohio and Mississippi Rivers in the spring of 1842 and painted a memorable scene of the raw, primitive frontier lifestyle made bleak and helpless by disease. Dickens's account was inspired by his visit to Cairo, Illinois, situated at the junction of the two rivers. "[W]e arrived at a spot so much more desolate than any we had yet beheld," he began in *American Notes*. There, "on ground so flat and low and marshy, that at certain seasons of the year, it is inundated to the house-tops, lies a breeding-place of fever, ague, and death." It was a "dismal swamp . . . teeming . . . with rank unwholesome vegetation, in whose baleful shade the wretched wanderers who are tempted hither, droop, and die, and lay their bones." Cairo was, in his summary, "a place without one single quality, in earth or air or water, to commend it."[4]

Dickens incorporated this vision into his novel about the adventures of Martin Chuzzlewit.[5] Here the benighted countryside serves as a metaphor for a particularly American hell. Chuzzlewit has traveled to the United States to seek his fortune, accompanied by his always cheerful servant, Mark Tapley. After meeting assorted ridiculous Americans, prone to braggadocio and bombast, the two men are conned into buying land in the thriving community of Eden, vaguely located somewhere downriver from the community wherein they are lodging. It is touted as "an awful lovely place, sure-ly. And frightful wholesome, likewise!" (p. 348). They hear some unsettling comments, though. One man, after carrying on about the danger of snakes on the frontier, denies that mosquitoes are a significant problem, saying that "there air some catawampous chawers in the small way, too, as graze upon a human being pretty strong; but don't mind *them*— they're company" (p. 343). Another tells Tapley, just as he is running to catch the boat, that "nobody as goes to Eden ever comes back a-live!" (p. 371).

Chuzzlewit and Tapley find in Eden a "dismal swamp," full of "noxious vapour" and "pestilential air." Upon their arrival at the primitive river landing, a man approaches them. "As he drew nearer, they observed that he was pale and worn, and that his anxious eyes were deeply sunken in his head." The man explains that "I've had the fever very bad, . . . I haven't stood upright these many weeks." When Chuzzlewit and Tapley inquire whether anyone could help them with their baggage, the man replies that his eldest son would help if he could, "but today he has the chill upon him, and is lying wrapped up in the blankets." As to the rest of his family, well, "[m]y youngest died last week." He has buried most of his family and friends, except those who have fled. "Them that we have here, don't come out at night." Tapley inquires of him, "The night air an't quite wholesome, I suppose." The settler answers, "It's deadly poison" (pp. 375–76).

Tapley, as usual, endeavors to put a positive spin on the situation. He sets up their cabin as comfortably as possible, then walks down to the riverfront to draw water. Around him, "[a] fetid vapor; hot and sickening as the breath of an oven, rose up from the earth, and hung on everything around; and as his foot-prints sunk into the marshy ground, a black ooze started forth to blot them out" (p. 378). As Tapley makes the acquaintance of the neighborhood, he finds that all are sickly, and many have lost family members and friends. There is "an air of great despondency and little hope on everything" (p. 515). In his cheerful way, Tapley passes it off as seasoning, for "we must all be seasoned, one way or the other. That's religion, that is, you know" (p. 380).

Chuzzlewit quickly falls ill. "He shook and shivered horribly; not as people do from cold, but in a frightful kind of spasm or convulsion, that racked his whole body." Tapley goes to a neighbor for help, who "pronounced his disease an aggravated kind of fever, accompanied with ague; which was very common in those parts, and which he predicted would be worse to-morrow, and for many more to-morrows." Opening a trunk in his own sparse cabin, the friend brings forth a medicine that has been of some help in his own fever bouts (p. 517). After several weeks Chuzzlewit recovers, but Tapley falls ill. In the structure of the novel, this seasoning time makes Chuzzlewit a less selfish young man and serves as a turning point for his fortunes. The two escape from the mires of Illinois and make it, happily, back to the civilized land of England.

There is little subtlety in Dickens's narrative. He damns a whole country, occupied in the East by fools, in the South by evil slaveholders, and in the West by people enfeebled by the very environment that he hears so often praised. Dickens went no farther south than Richmond, so he had no direct experience of the climate there. Frederick Law Olmsted of New York did, however, and his descriptions of the desolation frequently found throughout the southern states in the 1850s echo Dickens's image of Illinois. The people are boastful, lazy, and ignorant; the forms of travel are hideously uncomfortable; the food is awful. Olmsted's sojourn followed Dickens's by ten years, and the former had clearly perused the latter's work, for Tapley is mentioned in his narrative. What is striking, though, in comparing the two accounts, is how similar the South and the West sometimes sound—even the southern part of the East Coast, in Virginia and North Carolina. The lack of civilization as defined by both authors, the presence of squalid living conditions, and the apathetic enervation draw the two regions together. And malaria is a defining feature of both.[6]

Mark Twain likewise remembered a boyhood on the Mississippi River with malaria a common visitor. He wrote fondly of a swimming hole where he spent many hours cavorting, but qualified his own version of Eden: "Bear Creek . . . was a famous breeder of chills and fever in its day. I remember one summer when everybody in town had this disease at once. Many chimneys were shaken down, and all the houses were so racked that the town had to be rebuilt." With the hyperbole that typified his later writings, Twain went on to claim that the shaking was so bad that the landscape was altered: "The chasm or gorge between Lover's Leap and the hill west of it is supposed by scientists to have been caused by glacial action. This is a mistake."[7]

Less famous observers of the North American frontier repeatedly echoed these descriptions of widespread, debilitating malaria that darkened the frontier experience. One mid-nineteenth-century jingle about Michigan advertised its charms: "Don't go to Michigan, that land of ills; The word means ague, fever and chills."[8] Nearby Ontario was similarly plagued, from the late eighteenth century into the 1870s. Malaria thrived near the rivers and lakes that formed the region's crucial transportation routes.[9] All along the Mississippi and Missouri valleys, as well as up and down the West Coast, malaria was reported as arriving shortly after the first pioneers built houses and began to clear land for farming.[10] It was, as Tapley said, evidently a necessary part of the seasoning, part of the transition from wild to civilized.

How accurate were these portrayals of the nineteenth-century frontier? Dickens's observations were based on a brief trip, but a physician without any inherent antipathy to the country, after a thorough investigation, arrived at similar conclusions for the majority of the North American interior. Daniel Drake, the preeminent physician and medical educator of antebellum Ohio, studied the diseases of the area between the Appalachians and the Rocky Mountains in depth and published his findings in 1850.[11] Drake gave prominent place to what he termed autumnal fever, a complaint known variously as "bilious, intermittent, remittent, congestive, miasmatic, malarial, marsh, malignant, chill-fever, ague, fever and ague, dumb ague, and lastly *the* Fever."[12] From his descriptions it is clear that these terms encompassed *vivax* malaria, *falciparum* malaria, and probably typhoid and a host of other fevers as well. The mapping of the modern diagnostic term *malaria* onto Drake's label of *autumnal fever* remains inexact, but certainly there was significant overlap. Most probably *falciparum* malaria was part of this "autumnal fever" complex, as it generally occurred in the fall; *vivax* would have been less prominently associated with the fall months but could also occur then as well.

Drake, like Dickens, saw in the swampy lowlands near the region's great rivers the primary breeding grounds of autumnal fever. He blamed the frequent inundations caused by seasonal flooding for much of this problem, as well as the presence of multiple natural and artificial lakes and ponds. Drake's book had a long section exploring the causes of his autumnal fever, and he discussed the idea that bad air, or *malaria*, arising from putrefying animal or vegetable matter, as distinguished from airborne animalcules, spread the disease. Drake clearly defined *malaria* as a *cause* of autumnal fever, not as a synonym for it; it was "the poison that produces autumnal fever," acting in conjunction with heat and moisture.[13] Not until much later in the century did the term for the cause of this fever became the name of the disease itself.

Drake found his autumnal fever to be widely distributed in the Old Northwest, as well as in the more tropical regions of the South. In the more northern areas, the fever was much more likely to be a benign or simple intermittent, while farther south the mortality was higher, since the more malignant versions prevailed. Drake did not accord specificity to the various forms of autumnal fever; rather he saw them merging and transforming according to complex local conditions. Still, his account does support the likelihood that *falciparum* malaria was rare in the Ohio and upper Mississippi valleys, while *vivax* was common. His description of 3 to 5 percent mortality from the benign autumnal fever accords with twentieth-century observations of *vivax* malaria. It is here that Dickens was most off the mark, for he exaggerated the southern Illinois settlement's mortality rate.

Drake recorded other facets of frontier history that agree with modern knowledge of malaria. First, mosquitoes existed in large numbers on the frontier. One early French explorer of the lower Mississippi recorded in his journal that the "musketoes" made rest impossible and life miserable. "One is perfectly eaten and devoured. They get into the mouth, the nostrils, and the ears; the face, the hands, the body are all covered."[14] This plague of insects extended far north, into the icy Canadian wilderness. Dickens had a similar experience: on one occasion while meeting a dignitary in St. Louis, he commented that the fellow did not seem too impressed to meet the great writer, perhaps because of his casual clothing, "and my face and nose profusely ornamented with the stings of mosquitoes and bites of bugs."[15] Hence the mosquitoes were there, presumably including anopheles species, although observers made no such fine distinction.

But the generation of "autumnal fevers" required more than mosquitoes and people; the plasmodium had to be present as well. One would expect that initially the river settlements would be healthy, and that only over time would malaria appear. This is in fact what Drake described. The experience of a group settling near Peoria, Illinois, was typical. At first, "a number of families had settled (as is common) on the margin of a large prairie, and remained healthy in autumn." Then more people came and increased the amount of plowing around their cabins. By the second fall they "suffered severely in autumn from fever."[16] Another frontiersman living near Springfield told Drake that he had "resided where [Drake] found him three years, before a member of his family was seized with that fever." Drake was puzzled: "Such instances are not uncommon, though difficult to explain."[17] While contemporary opinion held that perhaps this resulted from turning up the soil and exposing poisonous sources of vapor, it is clear in retrospect that time was needed for the critical conjunction of people, parasites, and mosquitoes to converge on a given spot.

Drake's observations were echoed in the writings of frontier explorers and settlers. Historian Erwin Ackerknecht, whose study on malaria in the Old Northwest deserves its place as a classic in American medical historiography, provides abundant evidence of malaria and mosquitoes in the writings of settlers in such unlikely sites as Wisconsin, Minnesota, and Iowa.[18] More recently, Conevery Bolton has described the pervasive effect of malaria on life in Arkansas and Missouri in the first half of the nineteenth century.[19] Again and again lands that initially seemed wholesome became laden with periodic fevers, exhausting human capital. Malaria was added to the many dangers of the frontier—Indians, starvation, lawlessness, and rattlesnakes—to build an image of wildness and peril. But as civilization moved in, with its tighter houses, better-drained towns and fields, abundant food, and access to quinine, malaria receded. Everywhere, that is, except in the South, which in many ways retained a primitive, frontierlike culture well into the twentieth century.

Still, on the eve of the Civil War, physicians in Indiana, Ohio, and Illinois were just as familiar with the ravages of malarial fevers as were their colleagues in the southern and southwestern states. All were aware that quinine sulfate, first manufactured in the 1820s, was efficacious in cases of intermittent and remittent fever, although they continued to employ other remedies to "ready the system" for quinine, such as bloodletting, emetics, and purgatives.[20] In fact, southern physicians continued to administer the latter two treatments for malaria into the 1940s. So quinine was not seen as a specific for intermittent fevers—it was used for other fevers and as one of several remedies for intermittants—but we can at least say in retrospect that Civil War physicians had one tool in their armamentarium that did actively alleviate their patients' suffering.

The medicine that Tapley's Eden friend pulled out of his trunk was probably quinine, in the form of a patent remedy called Sappington's Anti-Fever Pills. John Sappington was a rural Missouri physician who had heard about the isolation of quinine from cinchona bark early in the 1820s. He rode off to Philadelphia, acquired a large supply, brought it back to Missouri, and began manufacturing a legendary product that may well have facilitated the growth of the American Midwest. Sappington's pills contained a grain of quinine, and he recommended 5 grains a day as a preventive and 8 to 16 grains a day for treatment. Over the next thirty years, Sappington sold nearly six million boxes containing twenty-four pills apiece. So quinine, in this and other forms, was widely available and familiar to patients and doctors alike on the eve of the Civil War.[21] Other patent remedies followed quickly on Sappington's heels, both incorporating quinine and offering alternatives to it. Quinine is unpleasant to take, given its bitter taste and unpleasant side effects of tinnitus and nausea. Drugs such as Thermaline ("A carefully prepared combination of the active principles of Calisaya Bark, and a species of the Fever Tree of Australia") which claimed to offer all of quinine's benefits with none of its side effects, also sold well.[22]

## Malaria in the Civil War

Not surprisingly, quinine was one of the most frequently used drugs of Civil War medicine. After various dysenteries and diarrhea, malarial fevers were the most common diagnoses in Union camp hospitals. The medical statistics compiled after the war for Union troops listed 1.3 million cases and more than ten thousand deaths from intermittent and remittent fevers.[23] Some of this infection happened to New England boys who met the malaria parasite for the first time in the boggy peninsular campaigns or in the battle for Vicksburg. Other Yankees hailing from the Old Northwest brought their own parasites along, allowing for a rapid spread of disease as the Union troops camped near mosquito breeding grounds throughout the South. Southern troops no doubt suffered as well, but the statistics for their morbidity and mortality are not systematically available.[24]

Midcentury physicians had the knowledge to reduce the impact of disease on troops, but the application of this knowledge was spotty at best. Contagious diseases like measles and smallpox were recognized as such and were dealt with by quarantine, movement of camp, and in the case of smallpox, vaccination. That the fecal filth generated by man and beast was connected to the onset of diarrheal diseases was widely acknowledged, even though the suspected source—poisonous vapors arising from piles of rotting manure—was not correct. Nevertheless, the enforcement of more thorough sanitation in camp and hospital, based on available knowledge, would have reduced casualties.[25] Finally, midcentury Americans knew how to avoid malarial fevers: stay two or three miles from the source of poisonous vapor, namely wetlands filled with rotting vegetation. Again, the etiology was wrong, but the prophylaxis effective.

This understanding that staying away from swampy areas was a way to avoid intermittent fever was not elite knowledge confined to physicians. A volunteer at Harper's Ferry in 1861 noted the "hopeless desperation chilling one when engaged in a contest with disease. The unseen malaria has such an advantage in the fight." His solution? "A week on a high piece of ground three miles from the river would put us all on our feet again." But he despaired of this simple solution, because the troops were needed to guard the river, not the land three miles away. So, he concluded, "as long as the morning sun rises only to quicken the fatal exhalations from this pestilential Potomac, and the evening dews fall only to rise again with fever," his comrades would remain cursed by fever and chills.[26]

The Union medical corps did try another way of preventing intermittent fever, which was to dose the men with quinine on a daily basis. All together the Union Army consumed almost 600,000 ounces of quinine sulfate and a similar amount of a cinchona extract. Although the doses were too low and irregularly given to do much to *prevent* malarial infection, they may have alleviated some of the debilitating symptoms. Quinine was dissolved in whiskey, to increase its appeal (and help hide its bitter taste), but most men preferred the whiskey alone. All told, quinine rations were not particularly successful.[27]

When soldiers returned from the Civil War, they started countless local epidemics of malaria at home, including areas not afflicted for decades. In New England, an epidemic ignited in the Connecticut River valley did not burn out until the 1890s. Not only did Yankee soldiers bring malaria home from the American South, but European immigrants imported malaria from Italy, Greece, and elsewhere as well. There were several outbreaks of malaria in New York City in the last half of the nineteenth century, probably due to the immigrant influence more than to the Civil War.[28] Ackerknecht's work shows that the parasite had a postwar boom in many of the states of the upper Mississippi valley, but by the first decade of the twentieth century, it had retired to the southern states. The exceptions were the southern tip of Illinois (site of Dickens's Eden), eastern Missouri, and western Kentucky, where malaria remained measurable into the 1930s.[29] Malaria also persisted in the central valley of California well into the twentieth century.

## Malaria Retreats to the South

Why did malaria largely disappear in the Old Northwest, where it had formerly been a major disease problem? And why did it not leave the South until five decades later? Although malaria had a major presence on the frontier in the mid-nineteenth century, it faded out in that region before measures based on an accurate knowledge of disease transmission could be implemented. In other words, malaria disappeared from the upper Mississippi valley without any active public health campaign against it. Writing in the early 1940s, Ackerknecht observed that malaria continued to thrive in the American South and wondered what critical differences between these regions had determined these outcomes. Ackerknecht was a historian, not a malariologist, but he drew on the works of contemporary specialists such as Mark Boyd, M. A. Barber, L. W. Hackett, and C. C. Bass in his examination of this question.[30]

Ackerknecht distilled the ideas of these various malariologists—a long list of potential factors—into a concise roster of possible explanations for malaria's disappearance from the upper Mississippi valley. He concluded that no one of them held the complete answer, but that several components of frontier life changed over the nineteenth century in ways that routed malaria. He was particularly interested in those lifestyle aspects that might be collected under the rubric of "increasing civilization": improvements in housing and food supply, drainage of the land, and increased access to physicians and medicine. Driven by a prosperous economy, settlers built houses that were more airtight to keep out winter's cold (and incidentally mosquitoes), drained land to expand their arable acreage for profitable crops (reducing mosquito breeding sites), and built a market economy that provided a steady supply of varied and nutritious foods. The most prosperous settlers screened their houses to keep out pests, without any direct knowledge that they were thereby avoiding disease. With rising prosperity more people could afford quinine, and the price of quinine also fell over the last decades of the nineteenth century, making it even more accessible. Quinine neither cured nor prevented malaria, but it did enable workers to get out of bed and go back to work, harvesting crops or otherwise maintaining the family's income. And quinine may have reduced the parasite burden enough to diminish disease transfer from one person to the next, although this effect would have been minor. All together, as the prosperity of the upper Mississippi valley made its environment less hospitable, malaria was less able to thrive.

Ackerknecht also examined whether the growing population of cattle and other livestock might have deterred malaria. Here he drew on the works of Rockefeller researcher Lewis Hackett. Hackett had explored the puzzle of "anophelism without malaria," a phenomenon in parts of Europe where anopheles mosquitoes feasted on people with abundance, but malaria did not occur. Hackett discovered that certain subspecies of the European malaria vector, *Anopheles maculipennis,* preferred to take its blood meals from animals rather than humans. Only if no animals were available would the mosquito choose human victims. So if livestock were present, they would divert the mosquitoes.[31] Drawing on this relatively new information (Hackett's book was only published in 1937), Ackerknecht posited that the growing numbers of beef and dairy cattle in the Old Northwest could have diverted American anopheles, reducing the number of human bites and breaking the chain of malaria transmission.[32]

Ackerknecht was also aware that as railroads were built throughout the area, population moved away from watercourses, the only previous source of rapid transportation. While he did not dismiss the importance of house location, he might have made more of the voluntary and deliberate nature of such movements. People did not just move toward the railroad; they moved away from areas they perceived as sickly. There was general knowledge that swamps and other stagnant waters were unhealthy, even if the assumed source of danger, swamp air, was falsely charged. Patent medicine advertisements played on this theme of wetlands as a fever source and informed any who were not aware that the night air off still waters could breed malarious fevers. For example, the J. C. Ayer Company of Lowell, Massachusetts, one of the most successful nineteenth-century patent medicine companies, advertised its "ague cure" on advertising cards that read "Malarial disorders . . . owe their origin to a miasmatic poison, which enters the blood through the Lungs, deranges the Liver, and causes the various forms of agues and fevers, and blood-poisoning." In case the audience was unclear about the origin of the malarial poison, the advertising copy was accompanied by a cartoon illustrating a cabin on the edge of a lake. Live oaks and palm trees, along with an alligator and frogs inset in one corner, make it clear that this is a bayou scene from the southern Gulf Coast. Carolina Tolu Tonic noted malaria's prevalence in the wet fields of rice cultivation, while Brown's Iron Bitters claimed, "Malaria['s] . . . cause is in most cases attributed to local surroundings, impure water and marshy ground." These advertising messages, all produced between 1870 and 1900, illustrate the popular understanding of malaria fevers as being generated by place and caused by the inhalation of bad air.[33] It is not at all inconceivable that the inhabitants of the upper Mississippi valley, inundated with such messages, deliberately moved their houses as far away as possible from dangerous wetlands (and not just toward railroad depots).

"Now, the eradication of malaria from the Upper Mississippi Valley was to a large extent the work of indirect measures undertaken without sanitary intentions: better agricultural methods, cattle breeding, better housing, screening, more prosperity, education, . . . [and] quinine," Ackerknecht summarized.[34] The important point here is that while many human actions changed the environment in ways that made malaria less likely to occur, few of those changes were made deliberately for the purpose of controlling malaria. Ackerknecht also stressed that no single effort brought an end to malaria, and that the risk remained (in 1945) that the disease could return to the area. "[I]t may be well to remember," he said in closing, "that malaria in the Upper Mississippi Valley was not killed by a single magic bullet; the monster was only put in chains. . . . Each link of the chain is important, and the breaking of one link may set free again the evil fiend."[35] At that time American malariologists were actively fighting malaria in the southern states and straining to prevent its reintroduction to multiple parts of the country by troops returning from disease-ridden war zones. Ackerknecht's struggle to assign proper weight to the different factors of disease causation and disappearance in the nineteenth century held common cause with the malariologists of his day, who were combating malaria in the United States and around the world.

## Medical Knowledge in Transition

Knowledge about the dangers of swamps, habitation near them, and night air was widespread. Some physicians were becoming dissatisfied with this explanation of intermittent fevers, however, seeing it as simplistic and incomplete. In the 1840s a transition in Western medical explanation began that prepared the way for the germ theory of disease and ultimately the understanding of the mosquito as a disease vector. Early nineteenth-cen-

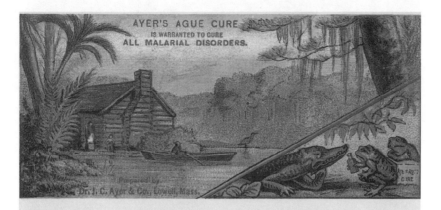

Ayer's Ague Cure. The Spanish moss, palm trees, flamingo, and alligator on this nineteenth-century advertising card all point to a Gulf Coast location, although for much of the century malaria was a problem of the temperate United States. Claiming to be quinine-free promised avoidance of quinine's unpleasant side effects, while the inclusion of typhoid recalls the common contemporary confusion of the two diseases.
(Advertising card in the author's possession)

tury European and American physicians commonly believed that fevers were fluid disorders. Although generated by exposure to foul miasms (which could arise, say, from rotting vegetable matter or animal excrement), fevers could be modulated by age, sex, climate, ethnicity, or season of the year. After physicians roughly localized a fever to an organ if possible (lungs, gut, joints, skin, brain), they classified it as mild or malignant, continuous or intermittent. Thus one disease could turn into another, as when a pneumonia turned into tuberculosis, or a mild dysentery "went into" cholera. This confusion was never absolute—smallpox was easily recognized as a distinct disease, for example—but the lack of specificity in categorizing infectious diseases limited understanding and research into cause and cure.[36]

This began to change by midcentury. After Asiatic cholera swept repeatedly over Europe and the United States between 1832 and 1865, almost all physicians recognized its identity as a separate and distinctively lethal disease. Medical researchers in the hospitals of Paris, who followed patients from clinic to autopsy, began to recognize distinctive pathological signs for such diseases as typhoid fever and typhus fever, and were able to correlate their discoveries with symptoms. German pathologist Rudolf Virchow used newly powerful microscopes to demonstrate the footprints of disease at the cellular level, driving an awareness that precise classification was possible. All told, physicians moved away from seeing diseases as fluid entities malleable by place and circumstance toward recognizing that there could be fixed disease descriptions, based on symptoms, physical signs, and pathological anatomy.[37]

This tendency toward greater specificity in disease classification led to a concomitant drive toward greater specificity in disease etiology. As long as physicians believed that local circumstances could transmogrify a fever into pneumonia or smallpox or cholera, it did not much matter what exactly set it off, and a vaguely defined miasm would suffice as a cause. But if typhoid fever could be distinguished from cholera and was a disease sui generis, then it needed its own distinctive etiology, separate from that of cholera. Simply blaming miasms arising from foul watercourses was not enough. What exactly was in that bad air that made people sick? One Charleston physician despaired in 1849, "The precise nature and composition of the noxious exhalations called technically miasma or malaria have never been discovered by the most skilful chemists."[38] Researchers looked for a specific component of the malodorous air that would be consistent with the overabundance of heat, moisture, and rotting substances that seemed to characterize miasms. Some explored the morbid qualities of hydrogen sulfide; others targeted heat and moisture themselves as causing disease. A few physicians speculated that suspensions of microorganisms, especially moisture-loving fungi, explained the matter. For example, John

K. Mitchell of Cincinnati argued that different species of fungal spores caused, specifically, yellow fever, intermittent fever, and cholera. On the other hand, Josiah C. Nott of Mobile published the theory, considered prescient by some, that tiny winged insects or animalcules floated in the miasmatic mists, each specific for a certain infectious disease.[39]

This discussion emerged largely in a climate of concern about cholera and yellow fever, two devastating epidemic fevers that demanded attention and explanation at midcentury. The arguments about their specific causes were tied directly to controversies about contagion. If cholera had a specific cause, then why was it present in some years (i.e., 1832 and 1848) but absent for decades at a time? Surely there were plenty of filth in the streets and plenty of miasms in the air in the meantime. The same argument applied to yellow fever: why was it sometimes present in filthy southern cities and not in others? One proposed answer was that the germ or animalcule or fungus was transported into the community, then thrived and reproduced in appropriately foul air.

Arguments about contagionism and transportability, however, were never relevant to malaria. Malaria tended to occur in the same places, year after year. No one even suggested that it might be contagious; it was too clearly tied to place, not person. By 1878 one Savannah physician could write with confidence, "It is pretty generally admitted, by medical scientists, both in America and Europe, that malarial or paludal fevers are produced by plants, or spores of plants, growing in marshes, stagnant water or elsewhere." He went on to admit that, "it would be impossible to say, whether those [plants] producing malarial fever belong invariably to the fungi order."[40] Leaving aside his confusion about fungi being plants, this physician clearly expressed the typical view of his day that malaria was tied to marshes, and that something that was growing in the marshes and that could be inhaled probably caused the disease.

In sorting out specific disease entities and their etiologies, intermittent fever was frequently compared to yellow fever. In particular, *falciparum* malaria was compared to yellow fever, since the two diseases shared a geographical and seasonal locale. Now known to be tied to the habitation and life cycle of mosquitoes, the occurrence of these two diseases from midsummer to first frost in areas of the hot humid South attracted questions about what they had in common. First to be sorted out was the issue of whether they were in fact separate diseases. Articles appeared comparing and contrasting the various symptoms and signs of the two diseases.[41] This distinction became of critical importance when yellow fever first appeared in a city. By the 1870s most physicians, government officials, and the lay public believed that yellow fever was contagious and could be stopped by quarantine. If it should arrive in one location, the best response was to use quarantine to contain it there. Naturally, quarantine harmed the commercial interests of a city, since it stopped trade, so those interests put pressure on local physicians not to reveal the presence of yellow fever. One common alternative diagnosis was malaria, as in "It's only a severe case of malaria. Nothing to be alarmed about. Not yellow fever at all." Multiple disputes over such sentinel diagnoses divided the public health officials of southern communities, especially those marked by commercial rivalries.[42]

During the 1870s a "new" disease appeared in the southern medical literature: hemorrhagic malarial fever. This form of malaria included a strong bleeding tendency, in which the patient produced bloody urine as well as black vomit, a cardinal symptom of yellow fever. When the esophagus or stomach lining bleeds, the resulting blood is turned black by gastric acid, resembling coffee grounds when vomited. Any disease process that causes upper gastrointestinal bleeding (like peptic ulcers and esophageal varices) can cause black vomit, but in the setting of a high fever and jaundice during a hot New Orleans summer in the nineteenth century, yellow fever had priority in the differential diagnosis. As a result, the claim that certain forms of malaria could become hemorrhagic became critical to public health debate. Leading the discussion was J. C. Faget, a New Orleans physician, who said that hemorrhagic intermittent fever had appeared for the first time during the 1853 yellow fever epidemic in New Orleans. "We saw the children, creole as well as stranger, *colored as well as white,* attacked epidemically with a fever, during which the black vomit was quite frequent." Faget concluded the disease could not be yellow fever, because it responded to quinine and was not deadly, whereas yellow fever, having reached that stage, would have behaved just the opposite.[43] While Faget garnered considerable support from other physicians who claimed to have seen his severe type of malarial fevers, in retrospect it appears that his critics were right that he was describing variants of yellow fever.[44] Some severe forms of malaria cause hemorrhage; another contender for this phenomenon is severe dengue. But this "hemorrhagic malaria" seems to have been too consistently tied to yellow fever epidemics to be a distinct etiology. In any event, the disease appears to have disappeared from the South along with yellow fever.

Another disease that emerged after the Civil War to confuse research on intermittent fever was typhomalaria. First described among Civil War soldiers by American physician J. J. Woodward in 1863, typhomalaria was distinguished by fever, extreme fatigue, headache, splenomegaly, and diarrhea. Woodward believed that typhomalaria was a specific disease generated by two separate causes—miasms from rotting vegetable matter and miasms from human feces and other animal wastes. Physicians found typhomalaria a useful label, for epidemic fevers often did not sort themselves into neat categories. British army surgeons stationed at Malta during the

1870s took up the designation for a fever raging in their camps that seemed to be linked both to poor sanitary conditions and to nearby malodorous marshes. Although some critics doubted the specificity of the new disease, it managed to survive challenges from microbiology in the 1880s and 1890s, when specific causes of both typhoid fever and malaria were identified. American army researchers put the matter to rest during the Spanish-American War in 1898. Armed with accurate diagnostic tools, they established once and for all the myriad presentations of typhoid fever and attached a relatively tiny role to malaria in characterizing an outbreak of what had been called typhomalarial fever. The men had typhoid fever, and camp sanitation, not quinine, was the necessary solution.[45]

During the last two decades of the nineteenth century, a great revolution in etiological thought occurred in medicine. By the 1890s the work of Robert Koch, Louis Pasteur, and their students had established that many diseases are caused by microorganisms. The first microbes suspected as disease agents were the fungi, for the action of yeast suggested analogically that such beings could reproduce explosively in human bodies and cause disease. Since certain diseases seemed to be correlated with heat, moisture, and filth, and fungi were observed to grow well in these conditions, the conclusion made sense that what was growing in all that humid putrescence was a fungal organism that caused disease. Not surprisingly, a fungus was "discovered" that caused yellow fever, and a fungus was sought to explain intermittent fever. This research plan proved a frustrating dead end, even though it correlated with the known distribution of these two diseases.[46]

During the 1880s bacteria came to the forefront as the principal suspects in infectious diseases. One after the other, the bacterial etiology of tuberculosis, cholera, diphtheria, and pneumonia was demonstrated. At the height of this bacterial excitement, a French physician in Algiers noted odd dark forms inside the blood cells of malaria patients. Could this be the causative organism? But the creature had many different forms, and it resembled debris more than any known bacterial cause, so when Alphonse Laveran proposed it as the cause of malaria, he was at first met with sneers of ridicule from the great modern minds of medicine. Koch doubted his findings, and the great Sir William Osler declared that he was seeing only detritus. Still Laveran labored away, trying to find his crescent-shaped beings in the soil and swamps of Algiers, with no success.[47] Others thought *they* had found the causative organism of malaria, and that it was a bacillus. Edwin Klebs, the codiscoverer of the diphtheria bacillus, and Corrado Tommasi-Crudeli claimed to have identified the germ in postmortem malaria cases, and they inoculated animals with it, creating new cases of malaria. Eventually their ideas faded, and by the mid-1890s most microbiologists accepted Laveran's organism as the cause of malaria. But like Laveran, they were stymied in trying to find its place in nature. Where did it live, and how did it get inside human bodies?[48]

A change in language coincided with this insight into malaria's etiology. Before the 1880s the word *malaria* had been used to refer to an aeriform poison, but it now came to mean the disease itself. One eminent New Jersey physician laid out this transition in 1886. "The word Malaria may be said to be in everybody's mouth," he began. "To the unprofessional mind, it means chill, aching bones,—creeping rigors,—and all, or either of the symptoms which announce the advent of fever," whatever its periodicity. Even physicians had used the term "in a vague and limitless meaning." He questioned whether "there is another word in the nomenclature of medicine, that is employed in such a careless and indeterminate sense as this single word,—*Malaria.*" He summed up the confusion with the revealing statement, "It passes current in professional circles, as denoting an invisible, intangible, undefined, and undiscovered cause for a variety of conditions, which are recognized as malarial, and which are diagnosed as malaria."[49] In the 1890s, however, as Laveran's germ gained in recognition, the old use of the term faded. No longer was malaria a poison but a disease caused by these dark, odd-shaped forms.

Some held tenaciously to the swamp poison concept, for how else could one explain the near-constant association of malarial fevers with low, wet, hot places? The strength of this correlation made acceptance of the mosquito theory overwhelmingly rapid. It was an amazing answer—Laveran's organism could be conveyed from person to person only by means of this winged pest, and that pest resided mainly in the vicinity of just those low, wet, hot places. Patrick Manson of England had suspected that mosquitoes explained malaria, after he had established that the tropical worm of filariasis was also carried by mosquitoes. He urged Ronald Ross, a student of his stationed in India, to find the means to establish the mosquito vector of malaria. In 1897 Ross did so, in birds. Italian researchers, furious at being scooped by this British colonial physician, rushed to prove that the anopheles mosquito was the vector for human malaria as well. The fact that their announcement in 1898 did not achieve the world acclaim (or Nobel Prize) that Ross's discovery inspired created a national antagonism in malaria research that persists, at least in humor, between English and Italian malariologists today.[50]

Robert Koch provided a further piece of the puzzle: the role of the malaria carrier and early concepts of malaria immunities. Koch studied malaria in the German colonies, first in East Africa and later in New Guinea. He paid little attention to traditional concepts of race and instead divided the world into two categories: the civilized German and the *Eingeboren,* the natives of a place. Thus he saw the black African and the light brown

New Guinea native in the same light—they were the native inhabitants of a malarious region, and as such a threat to the German colonists.[51]

Koch believed that malaria immunity was not genetic but primarily acquired. In communities with high malaria endemicity, he discovered, it was principally the children who became ill and who served to keep the malaria chain intact. The highest number of malarial illnesses was found in children, as well as the most deaths. Children had the greatest density of parasites in their blood. Adults, on the other hand, were rarely ill with malaria, even though parasites could be found in them. They were infected but not sick. Koch thereby concluded that the adults had acquired immunity by surviving the childhood disease experience. Nothing in his model suggested the concept of racial immunity; indeed, his very multiracial exposure may have argued against it, for who could say that the two native populations he studied were of the same race, in some sort of contradistinction to his own. Being an *Eingeboren* mattered; growing up in a malarious place mattered; race did not particularly matter.

Koch's work on malaria carriers dominated malariology in the United States and was firmly associated with his goal of eradicating carriers via the use of quinine.[52] A textbook about diseases of the American South, definitive for its time, illustrates the impact of Koch's work. After citing his New Guinea data, the authors agreed that immunity was acquired, not racially determined. They concluded that "the resistance of the black race to malaria is due to repeated attacks in early childhood, and not to any great extent to heredity."[53] Emphasis on acquired immunity highlighted the existence of adult carriers, while downplaying the race issue. Anyone could become an adult tolerant of malaria if they grew up in the right environment, so the link between the carrier state and race was much weaker than might be expected.

By 1900 the foundation was complete. Scientists knew the plasmodia by name and activity, the role of the anopheles mosquito, and how to fight that mosquito menace. This last part of the structure came from the work of L. O. Howard, America's great entomologist. Howard did experiments on the destruction of mosquito larvae, demonstrating that putting a thin layer of oil on top of their watery incubation sites would smother fledgling mosquitoes. After studying its effect on fish and other wildlife, he pronounced the oiling method safe. So there were now two basic tools for attacking mosquitoes—draining wetlands, and coating bodies of water with oil. In addition to these rudimentary techniques, Howard pointed out the usefulness of installing fine mesh screens in houses to shut out mosquitoes, burning mosquitocidal chemicals such as pyrethrum, and physically hand-killing adult mosquitoes.[54]

It was the yellow fever mosquito, whose viciousness was established by Walter Reed and his research colleagues in 1900, that first attracted the attention of public health officials. Campaigns in Cuba and New Orleans targeted the *Aedes aegypti* mosquito with the methods listed above, although the strategies had to be adapted to the preference of this mosquito for freshwater containers in urban settings. The most famous of such campaigns was carried out in the Panama Canal Zone, where American physician William Crawford Gorgas controlled both yellow fever and malaria, allowing the canal at long last to be built. Gorgas fought malaria with two weapons, quinine and antimosquito measures, thereby reducing its incidence by 80 to 90 percent. Knowledge of the mosquito vector justified older methods of malaria control (quinine, drainage, location away from swamps) and guided new actions, such as oiling wetlands to kill mosquito larvae. Public health officials throughout the United States were impressed by the campaign's success. Gorgas had shown that it was possible to conquer two great diseases.

But could it be done in the American South, which was now characterized as diseased, slothful, and mired in poverty?[55] Yellow fever, the terrifying disease that had stimulated so much federal and local public health activity targeting the South, proved surprisingly easy to eliminate using the new methods. After the epidemic in New Orleans in 1905 was brought under control by antimosquito measures, yellow fever never returned to the North American continent. Malaria, though, was not to be expelled until the 1940s. Why should the less malignant disease be so much harder to destroy? What was it about the South—its people, its topography, its political will—that made malaria such a persistent pestilence? The disease had once been a problem throughout the United States. Now, with the exception of remote California, it was an exclusively southern blight. It had once defined the very nature of the frontier; now it indicted the state of southern civilization. As the twentieth century dawned, the tools were in place for the deliberate eradication of malaria. The chapters that follow will explore why, in spite of such available technology, it took another half century for the last indigenous pockets of malaria to vanish from the United States.

# Chapter 3

# Race, Poverty, and Place

At the turn of the twentieth century, malaria was in retreat everywhere in the United States except in the South. Analyzing this phenomenon requires leaving the dynamic, feverish communities of the nineteenth-century frontier for the sharecroppers' torpid life on the South's plantations. From 1900 to 1950, the southern economy changed slowly, maintaining a population in the greatest depths of poverty, a population dragged down by malaria, tuberculosis, syphilis, and hookworm. Local and federal public health officials implemented programs for combating these diseases, with varying degrees of success. The region was America's economic embarassment, and its multiple diseases a blemish on the national escutcheon. Before we can answer the question "Why did malaria ultimately disappear from the United States?" we must ponder why it persisted so long in the states of the old Confederacy.

My own approach to malaria's twentieth-century American career is to argue that malaria has to be understood within a web of socioeconomic as well as biological influences. This topic is part of a broader debate on the causes of malaria and the best way to control it. Stating that malaria is caused by poverty, for example, implies that social welfare programs that improve socioeconomic status will also depress the malaria rates. That experiment had been tried in Italy, without success.[1] A caution is in order, however. It is tempting to see socioeconomic explanations as somehow more moral than ones based on, for example, insect behavior. Poverty is evil and should be condemned, goes this line of thought; any diversion of such condemnation should be seen as abandoning the cause of social reform and improvement. Yet it is a bit fatuous to expect that *every* component of disease ecology will be traceable to racial and class discrimination. The mosquito's behavior may be just as relevant. So may the use of insecticides, which are easy to condemn in this post–*Silent Spring* era but clearly have their place in this story. In understanding malaria's disappearance from the South in the 1940s, one has to consider many factors, and evaluations of their importance should be based soley on their degree of impact on the parasite's biography.

## Malaria's Ecology

Exploring the ecology of the parasite and its host vector is a good place to start in understanding when and why the parasite thrived in the American South. Several strains of anopheles mosquitoes are found in the continental United States, including *A. quadrimaculatus, A. punctipennis, A. crucians,* and *A. maculipennis.* (*A. maculipennis* can be broken down into subspecies, and some authors put *A. quadrimaculatus* as one of them; such distinctions do not materially change the analysis that follows.) *A. crucians* and *A. punctipennis* are southern anophelines capable of transmitting malaria under laboratory conditions but were rarely significant vectors in nature. Both strongly prefer animals as the source of their blood meals, which likely explains this anomaly. *A. maculipennis* is the mosquito of the northern tier of states, the Great Plains, the mountains, and West Coast. *A. quadrimaculatus* is the vector of the South and lower Midwest and was the most important actor in malaria transmission there in the twentieth century. *A. maculipennis* is easily diverted to animals, and Ackerknecht was probably right that such diversion was important in the Old Northwest.[2]

As the only significant malaria vector in the American South, *A. quadrimaculatus,* with its peculiarities and habits, becomes central to our story. In the 1920s and 1930s, once Lewis Hackett and his colleagues had shown that diversion of mosquitoes from humans to animals could significantly lower malaria rates, malariologists in the United States asked whether *A. quadrimaculatus* likewise preferred animal blood to that of humans. If it did, then "zooprophylaxis"—locating animals near humans—should work. Hackett pointed out that such a method argued for a pig under every bed rather than a net over it (leaving aside the question of a chicken in every pot).[3] Research on this issue was both ingenious and tedious. Following a method devised by J. B. Rice and M. A. Barber, mosquitoes were trapped from a location near animals, such as the area under a farmhouse located next to stables containing livestock. The insects were dissected to see if they had taken a blood meal. If so, through a precipitin test, the researcher could discover if the blood came from a cow, goat, horse, dog, human, or cat. (Although dogs were occasional bite victims, cat blood almost never showed up.) By varying the testing environment, entomologists could discover the preferential and possible meals of a particular type of mosquito. It turned out that *A. quadrimaculatus* was indifferent to host species: it would take blood from whatever warm body was nearby, be it mare, cow, or woman.[4] Since the South's principal malaria vector showed no strong preference, the increasing livestock population likely had little influence on southern malaria rates.

*A. quadrimaculatus* has peculiar behavioral characteristics. It breeds only in still water and prefers an alkaline pH. Females will not lay their eggs alongside streams or drainage ditches, unless congestion or drought has created pools where a watercourse formerly flowed. The larvae are concentrated on the edges of ponds, where there is little wave action, and debris protects the larvae from foraging minnows.[5] In the subtropical climate that characterizes most of the South, the mosquito becomes dormant in winter. It hibernates in trees, under houses, and in caves. If a mosquito is carrying malaria plasmodia when she retires for the winter, the organism rarely, if ever, survives long enough within the mosquito for her to be infective come spring.[6]

Lewis Hackett once remarked that it was remarkable that malaria spread in the United States at all. "The most astonishing thing about malaria, considering the chances against its successful transmission in nature, is the appalling amount of it in the world," he wrote.[7] Compared to the tropics, the months with temperatures high enough for both mosquito breeding and parasite development within the mosquito host are quite limited. Further, *A. quadrimaculatus* is not a very efficient malaria transmitter. Transmission depends on the density of carriers, the density of female mosquitoes, and access of the mosquitoes to the carriers. It also depends on gametocyte density, and the ease with which the mosquito takes in the infection. Research has shown that only a tiny percentage of bites result in vector infection. Once infected, a mosquito has to survive for one to two weeks, so that the parasite can mature in her body; only then is it ready to be injected into a new host. For transmission to occur, the mosquito has to take a blood meal from a human within two months. If she does not, the parasite usually withers and dies in the mosquito host. Breaking the chain of transmission should thus be possible without eliminating all *A. quadrimaculatus* and all malaria carriers. As a U.S. Public Health Service malaria worker said in 1924, "Malaria is an exotic in the United States; it is a tropical disease. It does not belong here and does not flourish in the U.S. except . . . under abnormal drainage and subnormal living conditions."[8] Malaria's conquest of the United States was far more tenuous, and easier to break down, than it was in more tropical climates.

Certain areas of the South were particularly hospitable to breeding *A. quadrimaculatus*, featuring the requisite "subnormal living conditions." The most notorious was the delta region of the Mississippi and Yazoo Rivers. Since the river bottoms had been converted to agriculture by the levees built in the late nineteenth century, a once totally swampy area was made partially habitable and yielded incredibly rich cotton-growing soil. Some swamps remained, of course, and the rivers were still prone to flooding in wet years, creating countless ponds as the floodwaters receded.[9] Kenneth Maxcy of the Public Health Service described it eloquently in 1923: "The Mississippi Delta . . . is particularly favorable to heavy production of anopheles quadrimaculatus. The flat 'river bottom' land is everywhere traversed by sluggish streams, with dendritic bayou connections forming innumerable cypress and sweet-gum swamps." Within this bayou country were located "great cotton plantations worked by thousands upon thousands of negro families living under conditions of maximum exposure to mosquito bites."[10] The land was just dry enough to farm, but wet enough to breed *A. quadrimaculatus* abundantly.[11]

The Atlantic coastal plain, made up of the lowlands of the Carolinas, Georgia, northern Florida, and Alabama, formed the eastern malaria belt. There the underlying ground rock was limestone, a soft base that could easily be eroded or undercut by water, creating multiple shallow ponds with an alkaline pH perfect for breeding *A. quadrimaculatus*. Such "lime sinks" were ubiquitous in the landscape; TVA malariologists working in Alabama found some counties with 150 sink ponds. Other areas in the South had enough water to maintain *A. quadrimaculatus* as well. Eastern Texas and Oklahoma in particular had their own environments suitable for breeding—and a significant malaria problem into the 1940s.[12]

## *Malaria and the Southern Economy*

More than one observer has noted that areas where cotton is grown tend to be the most malarious. Cotton was an intensive hand labor crop, and most cotton was grown on plantations where sharecroppers were clustered in shanties located on the most marginal land, which was likely to be swampy. Maxcy accurately described the connection between type of farming and malaria. "Conditions are adverse to free transmission of malaria where the farms are large, . . . as in hay farms and stock farms, requiring only a few employees with machinery to cultivate large tracts." On such farms he noticed that "the houses are likely to be far removed from each other and from the breeding places of anophelines." He contrasted this situation to that of the cotton plantation. "Where the type of agriculture is intensive, requiring many hand laborers, as in the raising of cotton, where the homes are close together and located in the rich 'bottom lands' near anopheline breeding places," malaria thrives. He concluded, "In the south there is a striking connection between malaria and the raising of cotton."[13] This relationship was caricatured in a 1923 cartoon about the Georgia State Board of Health's efforts against malaria. It shows a white farmer carrying a bale of cotton on his back. Sitting on the bale is a black man, asleep. On his head is a mosquito as big as a terrier. Labeled "The Southern Farmer's Burden," this cartoon was ludicrous in its overt assumption that white southerners were doing all the work, but apt in its awareness of the connection between cotton culture and malaria.[14]

Malaria was less a problem on the rice and sugarcane plantations of Louisiana and Arkansas, a fact that intrigued malariologist M. A. Barber.

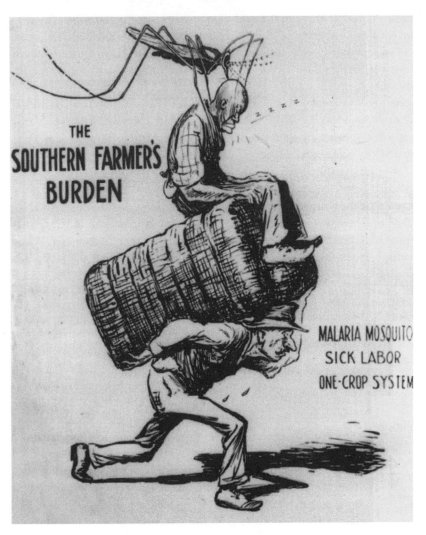

The Southern Farmer's Burden. In this 1923 USPHS cartoon, the white farmer is carrying the dual burdens of the fickle cotton economy and a black labor force enervated by malaria. The cartoon reflects the broader message that malaria blocked development and prosperity, and also the widespread assumption that blacks were disproportionately infected with malaria.
(Photographic Collection, Records of the USPHS, Record Group 90, NACP)

He explored this area in the mid-1920s and found *Anopheles quadrimaculatus* in great numbers. Like all rice fields, the ones he studied were crisscrossed with irrigation ditches and frequently submerged altogether. Various shelters amid the rice fields—such as outhouses, stables, unscreened dwellings, and even hollow trees—were blackened by the large number of mosquitoes roosting on them. He found one 12-by-13-inch board with 304 *A. quadrimaculatus,* while a colleague counted 2,768 in one barrel. So the right anopheles were there, and the people were there, but the malaria was much less substantial than on cotton plantations.

Barber explained this puzzle by using socioeconomic factors. Most of the rice field labor was done by machine, and no large rural population lived near the fields. More houses had screens in rice county, and the standard of living was generally higher. The sugarcane areas had concentrations of labor typical of cotton plantations, but much less malaria. When cotton areas typically had malaria rates of 8 to 10 percent, the sugarcane plantations only had 0.6 percent. This difference could not be explained by any public health interventions. Barber drew the following conclusion:

> It would seem that, with even a moderate betterment of social conditions, malaria in the U.S. tends to disappear or become relatively inconsiderable provided such improvement is general. Or, to state the proposition in another way, the maintenance of high endemic malaria requires a permanent reservoir of infection such as is furnished by a considerable body of people lacking proper housing, proper food, and adequate medical treatment. Now that pioneer conditions of life have in most parts of the country disappeared or become modified, it is usually a certain type of renter class which provides the necessary reservoir of infection. . . . It would seem that nearly every phase of economic improvement has had some effect on the reduction of malaria.[15]

In his 1946 autobiography Barber again told this story and still argued that what distinguished rice and sugar plantations was the relative prosperity of their workers. Moreover, in rice and sugar country, black farmhands lived in towns, rather than in "[t]he bedraggled huts so commonly seen along the bayous in cotton country."[16]

Where people lived was indeed critical to malaria prevalence, and the behavior of *A. quadrimaculatus* is important for understanding why. Whereas other mosquito species are likely to be found in barns or out in the woods, this mosquito tends to be found in houses. Hence it has easy contact with humans. After feeding, the female *A. quadrimaculatus* rests on a nearby wall (as opposed to flying outside), which makes it vulnerable to swatting or spraying. The mosquito rarely flies more than a mile from its breeding place, so in malarious areas the mosquitoes are densely clustered within a one-mile radius of ponds, while large swaths of drier land are visited only lightly. Malaria too is intensely local, so that in one county school 50 to 75 percent of students might be infected, while in another, in a higher, drier area of the same county, students might be much more sparsely infected. Malaria is not spread over an area like butter on bread but appears more like the currants in a bun, with foci of disease separated by healthy areas.[17]

So location was everything, and it was tied to economic conditions as well. Typically in untying the malaria knot, each aspect is connected to another. Such is the case with malaria and environment. Farmers who have adequate capital, producing a valuable crop, will drain as much of their land as possible to maximize the arable acreage. The affluent build their houses on high hills to catch the breezes and avoid mosquitoes; in the summer they send their children to vacation in the mountains to avoid the summer fevers. They can afford screens, quinine, and a doctor's care. Malaria is tied to poverty, but prosperity per se will not prevent or cure malaria. Gold coins laid over the eyes have no therapeutic value. Rather, it is possible and profitable to tease out just what it is that prosperity buys that wards off malaria.

As in most infectious diseases, malnutrition plays some role in immunity and resistance to malaria, but its role is difficult to quantify. The malnourished body may actually be less likely to get malaria, because it offers less sustenance to the invading parasite. The role of malnutrition in malaria has been discussed extensively, and one recent analyst has suggested that while chronic malnutrition is inimical to the parasite, episodes of acute starvation promote malarial deaths.[18] An indirect effect may be more important here than the direct impact on immune function during the acquisition of infection. The likelihood that a biting mosquito will pick up the gametocyte form of malaria from human blood—the only form that is ready in the mosquito's gut to continue the parasite life cycle—is correlated to immune adequacy. Malnutrition depresses immune function, increasing the likelihood that a malaria patient will have numerous gametocytes in his or her bloodstream. Thus a person's likelihood of getting malaria increases proportionately to the number of diseased bodies in the vicinity who are malnourished. As a corollary, the more such persons there are in one's home, the more chances exist for transmission to occur. The poor live more densely packed than the rich.

Similarly, comorbidities also influence immunity. Being sick with tuberculosis, hookworm, pellagra, or typhoid—all common diseases of the South's poor in the first half of the twentieth century—lowered resistance to malaria and encouraged gametocyte generation. Hookworm was particularly common in malarious areas, and some doctors even claimed that they could not cure a case of malaria until the hookworm was cleared as well.[19] Certainly pairing the anemia from hookworm with the anemia from malaria made for a very weak, sickly body. The same was true of tuberculosis, which also caused anemia, weight loss, and chronic disability. A woman worn out from repeated childbirth, whose body was sapped of iron and other nutrients, was an easy target for the malaria plasmodium.

Prosperity bought a decent house; poverty lived where it could. The "decentness" of a house could be defined in several ways. Its distance from swamps and ponds was key, and most people who could chose to live away from neighborhoods swarming with mosquitoes. A decent house had solid walls and floors; the sharecropper worried about rats and snakes entering through holes in the house, much less mosquitoes. Increasingly over the first few decades of the twentieth century, being prosperous meant having screens on windows and doors. Screens became an indicator of cleanliness and being middle class, though the issue driving screens was exposure less to mosquitoes than to flies. Anxious mothers feared the typhoid and polio carried on flies' feet, and increasingly an insect-free house became a sign of good housekeeping and hygiene. As early as 1915, the North Carolina *Health Bulletin* proclaimed: "Any home that would today be healthy or that has any idea whatever of decency will certainly have screens in the windows and doors of at least the dining room and the kitchen. The whole house should be screened."[20] In 1940 another author echoed this theme: "Screening is so much a matter of course in middle and upper-class homes and places of evening assembly in this country that we nowadays take it entirely for granted."[21]

Home insecticides became another common aspect of sanitary home treatment in the 1930s. Most widely used were kerosene solutions of pyrethrum, a powder made from a chrysanthemum indigenous to Dalmatia. Although pyrethrum powder had been burned for centuries to kill insects, the spray solution first became available for the domestic market after patent litigation in the 1920s released it for general production. The most common brand name was Flit, dispensed out of barrel-shaped sprayers with a plunger. Dr. Seuss illustrated advertisements for Flit, which all carried the punchline "Quick Henry, the Flit." The "Flit gun" became a common household implement, at least in middle-class households, and by 1935 pyrethrum imports exceeded 16 million pounds. Pyrethrum is a "knockdown" insecticide: it kills on contact but its toxicity wanes in a few hours. Still, studies in India in the 1930s showed that regularly killing adult mosquitoes with pyrethrum led to reduced rates of malaria transmission. Malariologist Paul Russell, for one, attributed some of malaria's decline in the United States to the ubiquity of domestic pyrethrum, saying in 1955 that "[s]ince 1930 hardly a house in the formerly malarious area [of the South] has been without its 'flit gun.'"[22] This was not likely true for the sharecropper's shack, but by the 1940s home insecticides, like screens, had become a common feature of middle-class homes.

In a sense this discussion about prosperity as a cause of diminished malaria is a subset of the broader debate over how much weight to attribute to housing, food, and comorbidities, and how much to attribute to medical practice. Did it matter that the affluent had access to doctors, hospitals, and medicines? Quinine was not an effective public health measure, but it did save lives on the individual level. The children of the affluent were not likely to die of malaria, but the infants of the poor might well do so. The poor tended to resort to self-medication with patent medicines such as Grove's Chill Tonic which promised effective quinine in a palatable form for infants. Yet the amount of quinine in chill tonics was rarely sufficient to make a serious dent in the disease. One physician found a young boy swarming with parasites—yet the boy had consumed three bottles of Grove's Chill Tonic in previous weeks.[23] The affluent who were ill with malaria, by contrast, got sufficient quinine, food, and nursing care, were kept in screened rooms, and had access to opioid analgesics to make the pains easier to bear. Since mortality was not the main issue in malaria, the doctor's presence and the ability to buy medicines would have had a greater impact on general health and well-being (although it did reduce mortality as well). But did medical care either reduce the transmission of malaria or limit it as a communitywide disease? Without knowing the answer, the impact of medical attendance on malaria rates remains unclear.

## Race and Malaria

What impact on malaria's prevalence in the South did the disproportionate percentage of southerners with African-American heritage have? The antebellum argument that slaves were appropriate for work in the South because of their immunity to malaria is well known. But what happened to this argument after the war? Did having a large black population make the South less prone to malaria, or more?

Between the 1890s and the Great Depression, discussions of the health of black Americans turned on two questions. Were they as a race declining to extinction? Were they a threat to the health of white Americans? The first, if answered positively, lent credence to the argument that blacks were better off under slavery and unfit for free society; the second, if answered positively, raised fears of racial contamination in the home, for blacks toiled in close intimacy to white families, cooking their food, cleaning their houses, and nursing their children. Curiously, while malaria carriers were recognized as a danger, they were not prominent in discussions about the health relationship between black and white Americans.

The most prominent voice proclaiming the imminent demise of the African race in America was Frederick Hoffman, an analyst for the Pru-

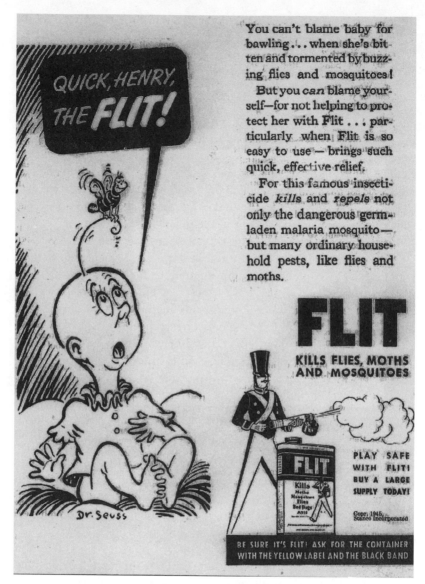

Quick, Henry, the Flit! One of a series of cartoons drawn by Dr.
Seuss for a popular brand of pyrethrum-based insecticide, this ad
plays on parental guilt about both mosquitoes and flies, known to
be important carriers of the typhoid bacillus. By 1945 enjoying a
mosquito- and fly-free home had increasingly become part of the
middle-class standard of living.
(Advertisement from unknown magazine, 1945, in the author's
possession)

dential Life Insurance Company. Hoffman, born in Germany, claimed in the preface to his 1896 treatise on health and race that he could be impartial on the subject because he had grown up with no inborn prejudices whatever.[24] His argument was that since the black population growth rate was only about half of the white, and the black experience of early disease mortality was growing, then the race was doomed to extinction in the United States. However self-congratulatory Hoffman may have been about reaching this conclusion, his racism shines through in comments such as, "The whole history of Anglo-Saxon conquest and colonization is one of endless proof of race superiority and race supremacy," as well as his assertion that "the rate of increase in lynching [in the American South] may be accepted as representing fairly the increasing tendency of colored men to commit this most frightful of crimes [rape]."[25]

Degeneracy was a major theme of *fin de siècle* sociology. Proponents of eugenics harped on the decline of the American breeding stock due to the influx of supposedly inferior immigrants, not to mention the sort of racial intermingling that was evident in the many lighter-skinned, Anglo-featured blacks in the United States. Fear of degeneracy fueled campaigns to sterilize the mentally deficient, whether their blight was insanity or low intelligence. Such thinking shored up the legitimacy of Jim Crow laws, for certainly everything should be done to keep the races separate to avoid that most dreaded of interactions, miscegenation, which would further weaken the stock.[26]

Hoffman's statistics also supported racist ideology that portrayed the black as helpless, shiftless, and unable to maintain his or her health and well-being without guidance from white masters. After claiming that blacks were too ignorant to care for their children properly, Hoffman went on to blame the higher mortality rates of African-Americans on another innate racial characteristic. "For the root of the evil," he claimed, "lies in the fact of an immense amount of immorality, which is a race trait, and of which scrofula, syphilis, and even consumption are the inevitable consequences."[27] Antebellum defenders of slavery had proclaimed that the black slave was like a child, in need of sustenance and discipline from the more mature white race. The infamous census of 1840, which purported to show that free blacks had high rates of insanity (unlike contented, mentally stable slaves) had been grist for this mill. Hoffman's work followed in this tradition of using statistics to demonstrate the inferiority and proper subjugation of black Americans. Certainly many racists were cheered by the thought that black health would so degenerate that the race would disappear.[28]

Nearly two decades after Hoffman's treatise appeared, however, it was obvious that the black population was not fading obligingly away, but rather was continuing to grow, albeit at a slower pace than whites. Disease rates were markedly higher among blacks, especially for tuberculosis and other respiratory ailments, and so were death rates. But given its compensatory birth rate, the population was not dwindling. Medical pundits, aware of these statistics, turned increasingly to seeing the black population as a direct threat to whites. "The Negro a Menace to the Health of the White Race," proclaimed the title of one typical 1916 article in the *Southern Medical Journal*.[29] Two infections drew most of the attention of this and other medical authors: tuberculosis and venereal disease. Tuberculosis was by then the subject of major public health campaigns, which focused particularly on teaching the patient to avoid infecting others by managing his or her infectious sputum properly. Venereal diseases were known to be a consequence of intimacy, but there was also fear that they could be transmitted through more casual contact.

Experts repeatedly warned about the proximity of the races. "We in the far South cannot afford to ignore the problem of the health of the negro," said one white New Orleans physician. "Negroes cook our meals, serve us at table, clean our houses, make our beds, launder our clothes, care for our children, in short, live in intimate daily contact with us and our families."[30] Another physician noted that the "negro health problem" was one of the "white man's burdens" because "[t]he white race and the black race will continue to live side by side in the South, and whatever injuriously affects the health of one race is deleterious to the other also." He was particularly concerned about venereal disease, because black women were "known" to be so ignorant, indifferent, and immoral. "Many negro women have gonorrhea, and pay little attention to it," he asserted. "This is a very real menace to our white boys, and through them, after marriage, to our innocent daughters also. For, despite our best efforts, many boys are going to sow wild oats."[31]

Tuberculosis and venereal disease were at the center of discussion at a 1914 meeting of health officers from the southern states on the subject "The Negro Health Problem." Oscar Dowling, head of the Louisiana State Board of Health, organized the meeting and served as its president. Representatives from every southern state board of health arrived in New Orleans to consider the "health of the Negro," "the most important single element in our problem of sanitary betterment." Much of the discussion concerned the role of poor housing in creating and maintaining disease. Although many no doubt agreed with the South Carolina physician who argued that only lazy, wastrel, and indifferent blacks lived in bad housing, which he said was all that they deserved, other voices called for landlords to take responsibility for the quality of their rental properties. The meeting allowed a group of black physicians to speak, and their message focused on the need for better housing and better health education for black people. Throughout this extensive discussion, tuberculosis and venereal diseases remained center stage; malaria was nowhere to be found.[32]

If black people were seen as such a source of infection, why wasn't the black malaria carrier a concern? The absence of malaria from these discussions demonstrates clearly that in the early twentieth century, the link between malaria and race had been considerably weakened.

The idea that malaria could be spread by carriers, apparently healthy individuals circulating in society, emerged only in the first decade of the twentieth century. Its conception depended on knowledge of the plasmodium and the mosquito vector, and that knowledge was in place as physicians began to design campaigns to control malaria. The earlier notion, that malaria was caused by a miasm emanating from swampy lands, made the potential victim fear a place, not a person. But now the infected individual was an essential part of the malaria chain, which linked victim to victim via the mosquito. Bacteriological studies of other diseases, such as diphtheria and typhoid, had shown that healthy people could spread disease without any outward sign of their infectivity. Typhoid Mary, an Irish cook in New York who shed typhoid bacilli in her stools but appeared robust and well, was the most famous. Researchers also discovered that the infected could be moderately ill but still up and about, serving equally well as transports for organisms. Tuberculosis was particularly notorious in this regard, and fear of the person who coughed on the train or spit on its floor grew accordingly. So malaria researchers were not completely taken by surprise when they found adults at their regular work with parasites abundant in their blood.[33]

German bacteriologist Robert Koch did much of the research on malaria carriers, as he had done for carriers of typhoid, tuberculosis, and other diseases. Koch, as we have seen, tended to divide inhabitants of the tropical communities that he studied into locals and foreigners, and he particularly worried that the locals were carriers and hence dangerous. He was less interested in a person's race than in where he or she had been born and raised. Koch saw almost all immunity in malaria as due to acquisition of protection over time after multiple exposures to the parasite. Race, and the idea of inborn characteristics, were not important to his understanding.[34] His outlook was widely accepted by malariologists in the United States.[35]

Interest in malaria carriers seems to have emerged and then faded with the rise and fall of quinine as a public health measure. This method, also tied to Koch's pronouncements, remained popular in the United States into the 1920s. Louisiana physician C. C. Bass promoted quinine therapy as a method of eradicating the carrier state and preventing relapse as well, frequently mentioning the importance of the carrier.[36] But once quinine was abandoned in favor of attacks on the mosquito, the carrier became rare as a topic in malaria control discussions. So while blacks were feared as transmitters of tuberculosis and venereal disease, their danger as malaria sources was not considered in the "Negro Health Problem" literature.

## Blacks and Malaria

Perhaps the major reason that blacks' supposed immunity to malaria faded from white consciousness was the fact that in the early twentieth-century South, a great many blacks had malaria. Over and over again mortality statistics showed more blacks than whites dying of malaria, often in ratios as high as two to one. U.S. Public Health Service researcher Kenneth Maxcy, for example, found twice as many cases of splenomegaly (a sign of malaria) among black Mississippi Delta schoolchildren as among white.[37] This difference was also borne out in studies that looked at parasite rates between the races. Although these statistics may have had various biases, public health officials, and the public at large, nevertheless clearly saw the black population as more at risk for malaria than the white. Table 1 shows parasite rates found in multiple surveys of black populations, especially black schoolchildren, and where available of whites.[38] When researchers compared black and white, blacks usually exceeded the parasite rates of whites. At certain sites as much as 42 percent of the black population was infected. Of course such percentages are very much dependent on the population surveyed, but these results at least indicate that public health researchers had no problem finding abundant malaria infestation among southern blacks.

Mortality rates, while less reliable than parasite surveys, also showed the greater prevalence of malaria among blacks than whites. Statistician Mary Gover summarized the data from the annual vital statistics gathered by the federal government from the state boards of health in papers published after World War II. She found that the comparative malaria death rate per hundred thousand people between black and white was at times as divergent as 22.4 to 1.9 (1919–21) and 5.6 to 0.6 (1939–41). The distance between the races remained remarkably constant, even as cases were declining in number for both.[39]

Discussions of this phenomenon reveal much about prevailing medical attitudes toward race and malaria. Some commentators said that if blacks had previously been somewhat immune to malaria, they had lost that protection now. Others explained that the prevalence of malaria among African-Americans had nothing at all to do with race but merely served as a marker of their socioeconomic status. And as always, questions arose about the validity of the data itself.

Arguments about blacks' loss of immunity drew explicitly on Koch's work. Those who maintained that blacks must have lost some protection

Table 1: Malaria Parasite Rates in the South

| Observer | Place | Year | Population Surveyed | Number | Percent Positive |
|----------|-------|------|---------------------|--------|------------------|
| Mitzmain | Scott, MS | 1915 | black sharecroppers | 1,184 surveyed | 42.0 |
| von Ezdorf | multiple sites in AL, AK, MS, NC | 1912–15 | black and white | 13,500 surveyed | 13.3 |
| von Ezdorf | multiple sites in AL, AK, MS, NC | 1912–15 | blacks whites | 5,607 7,893 | 20.6 8.1 |
| Taylor | Pamlico Co., NC | 1923 | black and white general population | not given | B 37.0 W 32.0 |
| Hass/Derivaux | Lake Village, AK | 1916 | black sharecroppers | 430 surveyed | 16.0 |
| Barber | multiple southern sites | 1924 | general population | 4,535 pos. smears | B 54.0 W 46.0 |
| Bass | Bolivar Co., MS | 1916 | black sharecroppers | 31,459 surveyed | 22.2 |
| Underwood | unspecified MS Delta | 1925 | black sharecroppers | 72 survyed | 17.0 |
| Griffitts | Dougherty Co., Georgia | 1930 | black and white rural schoolchildren | 334 surveyed | B 42.9 W 4.5 |

offered two strains of analysis. The first posited that since all immunity was acquired, the person who was not exposed frequently would lose protection. So if malaria declined in frequency, the continuous infection that had once produced an immune black adult was disrupted, leaving him or her just as susceptible to the disease as whites in colonial South Carolina had been. For example, Julian Herman Lewis argued in 1942 that "[t]here is no evidence that race per se is a factor in the existence or perpetuation of malaria." He admitted that "it has long been thought that the Negro is immune to the disease, the basis for which is the well-known fact that white settlers in parts of Africa where malaria is endemic rapidly succumb to the disease, while the natives flourish." Lewis explained this apparent immunity by noting a curious paradox—Africans were both heavily infected with parasites yet seemingly well. A black person's race did not determine immunity per se, for black children were badly afflicted with the disease. Rather, adults acquired immunity through long exposure. If immunity against malaria had declined among blacks in the United States, it was because they no longer had the protective effect of constant infection from infancy on.[40]

A second argument tied into the general theme of degeneracy. Proponents of this line of thought argued that just as blacks had not had tuberculosis to a significant degree before the Civil War, they also had not had malaria. Whether this was due to the good care they received at the hands of plantation masters or to some biological tendency was not always elaborated. Clearly, however, the black race had degenerated in freedom, they said, and now was sickly—sick with tuberculosis, sick with venereal disease, and sick with malaria. Their very degeneracy as a race set them up for this weakened state of affairs, it was said. Frederick Hoffman expressed this view clearly when he opined that "the tendency of the colored race towards a higher death rate and disease prevalence from malaria, is of comparatively recent origin," and "is in marked contrast to the lesser susceptibility of the white race." He attributed this to a nonspecific decline in "vital resistance" and tied it to the overall degeneracy of the black race in freedom.[41]

But more sympathetic observers of the high malaria rate in blacks attributed it to their socioeconomic status. Black southerners lived in porous houses on swampy land, which exposed them to many mosquito bites. The housing was crowded, both in terms of the occupancy of each cabin, and in the houses' proximity to each other, allowing for easy malaria transmission. Southern blacks were malnourished and overworked, making their general resistance low. And they lacked access to medical care, without money to pay doctors or buy medicine. These factors fed upon themselves, for they made not just malaria but other infectious diseases such as tuberculosis more likely, lowering blacks' immunity in general. Malaria was a marker of poverty, and advocates of this point of view believed that affluent southern whites should be ashamed that they allowed African-Americans to exist among them in such dire straits.[42]

A third response to the statistics was to examine the quality of the data itself. Were blacks more likely than whites to be labeled with malaria as a cause of death? Probably: when a team of public health officials reviewed the malaria death statistics in 1925, they found much reason to doubt the accuracy of malaria as a cause of death in general. More importantly for the current discussion, they discovered racial differences in malaria mortality reports. In the coastal counties of South Carolina, for example, many deaths occurred without the presence of a physician, and when the local registrar came to put down a cause of death, he or she had to guess, based on what the relatives said. Of these unattended deaths, 11 percent were called typhoid, 17 percent tuberculosis, and 50 percent malaria. That was for black people. But only 13.6 percent of the white deaths that went unattended were attributed to malaria. In two South Carolina counties that had the highest death rates from malaria in the United States, only 4 of 95 deaths from malaria had been certified by a physician.[43]

By and large, though, black Americans most likely suffered from a disproportionate burden of malaria. Their very ability to tolerate the organisms, both from acquired and inherited immunities, meant that the mosquitoes, which swarmed in the crowded sharecropper cabins, had a high rate of infectiousness and continued the malaria chain into the next generation. In spite of having some biological protection against the disease, black southerners undoubtedly suffered mightily from it well into this century. Their protection was far from absolute, as was transparent to medical observers.

Why did the very prevalence of malaria among black people not cause whites to fear them as a source of disease? The answers to this are complex and highly speculative. Blacks were not silent carriers, as Typhoid Mary had been, since they so evidently suffered from the disease themselves. For the black adult who was swarming with parasites but working in proximity with whites, the mosquito vector was less commonly available to transmit the parasite between them. Through mosquito control, malaria had been eradicated from most southern towns by the mid-1920s. Townspeople would have had less reason to fear a carrier when the vector, and the disease, appeared so diminished. Malaria was not like tuberculosis, spread by the wayward cough, or venereal disease, transmitted through the open sore. The requirement of the mosquito perhaps sheltered the functioning black worker from appearing to be an immediate source of disease. The black child, more evidently sick with malaria, would due to his or her very childishness be nonthreatening. Finally, the general focus on the mosquito, and inattention to the carrier, would deflect fear from the malaria patient. Whatever the reason, southern blacks acquired the reputation as victims of malaria rather than purveyors of it.

While various commentators thought the prevalence of malaria among southern blacks was worthy of comment, the notion that black people were somehow privileged with immunity to malaria seemed put to rest. Not until the 1930s did the notion of a racial immunity again surface in American medical thought. At that time this fact emerged from an odd source of therapeutic research: the use of malariatherapy for treating neurosyphilis.

## Malaria, Syphilis, and Race

A curious chapter in the history of malaria spans the three decades from 1920 to 1950. Physicians who were treating syphilis had been pleased that Paul Ehrlich's "magic bullet," salvarsan, had shown effectiveness in treating syphilis, even though the course of therapy was long and difficult. One component of syphilis remained stubbornly indifferent to salvarsan therapy, however—the infection of the central nervous system with the syphilis spirochete, called neurosyphilis. In the 1910s physicians began to note the odd fact that symptoms of neurosyphilis, such as dementia and partial paralysis, improved after the patient suffered from another disease that generated high fevers. They built on that observation by trying to design therapy that would intentionally generate a benign but high fever and thus help control the crippling neurosyphilis sequelae. Various methods of inducing fever were tried, including vaccines, infection with the erysipelas germ (a streptococcus), and finally malaria parasites.[44]

So successful did malariatherapy appear to be for neurosyphilis that in 1927 its designer, a Viennese physician named Julius Wagner von Juaregg, earned the Nobel Prize for his discovery. Soon physicians throughout Europe and the United States were using malariatherapy for their patients with severe neurological side effects from syphilis. These patients included a significant percent of inhabitants of mental hospitals and asylums, providing an ample population for research on the new technique. Physicians considered malariatherapy to be "standard of care" for neurosyphilis until after World War II, when penicillin became widely available for its treatment and slowly replaced the more dangerous and difficult use of live malaria parasites.[45]

The organism of choice for malariatherapy was *Plasmodium vivax. Vivax* caused very satisfactorily high fevers, was rarely a risk to life, and could be controlled with quinine. Ideally, the infection was transferred into the syphilitic via mosquitoes, which helped to filter out other possible impurities from the donor's malarious blood, although at times blood was taken directly from the donor and injected with a hypodermic. This mode of therapy was not without problems. It called for ingredients that might be difficult to find: a donor had to be identified and then paid not to take treatment so that his or her bloodstream could continue to provide parasites. If mosquitoes were used, they had to be bred and maintained in cages to avoid contamination with outside strains of malaria or other diseases. And there was always the danger that the malariatherapy might prove too toxic for the patient.[46]

These problems are all revealed in the notebooks that Rockefeller researcher and malariologist Mark Boyd kept about his use of malariatherapy at a mental hospital in Florida, along with a further issue. When Boyd and his colleagues tried to infect black syphilis patients with *vivax* malaria, the results were disappointing. The patient might develop a slight malaise and low-grade fever in response to the injection, but certainly not the high spiking fever that was required for the syphilis therapy to be successful. Boyd tried increasing the dose, but that did not help. He checked to be sure that his mosquitoes were actually "loaded," and that the parasites were present in the blood of the recipient. Everything about the technique was fine—but his patients did not become ill with malaria. He had proven, serendipitously, that many African-Americans were immune to *vivax* malaria. The explanation, based on the Duffy antigen, did not come until 1975, but the fact was thoroughly established through the research of Boyd and others in the 1930s. Boyd was able to infect his black patients with the much more dangerous *Plasmodium falciparum*, showing that they were not immune to infection with this parasite.[47]

It remained for A. C. Allison, in 1954, to postulate the connection between sickle-cell hemoglobin and partial protection from *falciparum* malaria. This work had nothing to do with malariatherapy for neurosyphilis, but instead grew out of his puzzlement about the overlapping distribution of high rates of sickle-cell disease with high densities of *falciparum* infection. He found that in parts of the world where malaria was hyperendemic (i.e., always present and causing high numbers of cases), the prevalence of sickle-cell trait was usually above 20 percent, and sometimes as high as 40 percent. But in areas of sub-Saharan Africa where malaria was sporadic, the sickle-cell trait appeared in less than 10 percent of the population. Allison further found that children with sickle-cell trait had a lower density of malaria parasites in their blood, and a greater chance of surviving to age five. Others later confirmed Allison's initial hypothesis, making the case of malaria and sickle-cell a classic instance of balanced polymorphism, a genetic phenomenon in which the heterozygous state of a particular trait is preferred over both the homozygous state and the absence of the trait.[48]

Tracing the complex course of southern whites' conceptions about black malaria immunity requires seeing both the underlying biology and the tendency of people to use science to argue the things they already believe. Arguments about blacks' abilities to survive in the tropics and function there as workers certainly had a phenomenological basis. They were biologically more suited to the sort of climate in which they had evolved for centuries and in which malaria had been a companion for generations. Once recognized, however, this fact was used by white southerners to justify slavery, arguing that enslaved blacks were well off as they were and where they were. After the Civil War, the pressure for this argument disappeared, and in its place grew an "I told you so" attitude that gloried in the unhealthiness of now-emancipated black southerners. Even as this attitude was replaced by general fears of contamination from tuberculosis and veneral diseases, malaria remained out of the limelight in discussions of race.

Malaria might well have been categorized with venereal disease and tuberculosis as threats of contaminating contact, if the personal contagion aspect of the disease had been more pronounced in the public health gospel. But after the interest in quininization and carriers faded with the failure of Bass's public health plan, the mosquito moved to the forefront of the public health malaria campaign. There simply was not much use for the race card in discussions of mosquitoes, and if anything the levels of malaria among blacks provoked discussions of their shoddy housing (leading to mosquito exposure) rather than fears about carriers. The housing issue cast a bad light on white property owners and pricked the communal social conscience; it did not raise concerns about personal infection, particularly after malaria disappeared from southern towns in the 1920s.

When information about racial immunity to malaria emerged in the 1930s, it served no propagandist issue. The focus was on the mosquito, and that preoccupation continued with the DDT campaigns of the 1940s. By the time Allison identified the sickle-cell phenomenon and its relation to malaria in the 1950s, malaria was largely of historical interest in the United States. Knowledge of malaria immunities would be useful for historians such as Philip Curtin, Peter Wood, and Ken Kiple in understanding the New World's history, but it had little relevance to the domestic public health effort in the United States.

Malariologist Marshall A. Barber summed up malaria's racial connections in the history of the United States in a particularly compelling passage of his autobiography:

> Negroes have long served as reservoirs of malaria parasites. Although perhaps suffering less from an attack of the disease than do white persons, they are probably quite as easily infected, certainly by the estivo-autumnal form of parasite. As a rule, Negroes are less protected from mosquito bites; and since they are more often neglectful of treatment, they are likely to harbor the parasite for long periods of time. Of course, any neglected people will serve as a reservoir of infectious disease. But with respect to malaria, Negroes are a particularly efficient reservoir or at least have been in the past. Equatorial Africa is stocked with species and strains of malaria parasites in great variety and abundance, and thousands of Negroes must have been loaded with them when the ships of the "middle passage" brought the Negro slaves to the Americas. There they remained an abundant source of infection, a menace to their former masters many years after slavery was abolished. Thus the Dark Continent avenged itself for the theft of its children.[49]

All together, in assessing why the South was peculiar in its holding on to malaria, multiple factors are important. It retained its frontier quality, with poor housing located near swampy land. It contained a large population of African-Americans who supplied a steady reservoir of *falciparum* malaria parasites. It contained a population that lacked adequate medical care or access to insecticides, and it had an inadequate tax base to support government programs. All of these factors contributed to the persistence of malaria in the South. These social, racial, and geographic aspects proved a mighty hurdle for the poorly funded public health infrastructure of southern states to overcome.

# Chapter 4                          Making Malaria
                                     Control
                                     Profitable

The first decades of the twentieth century were a time of great hope and
excitement about the possibilites of public health. Diphtheria, the child-
killing horror that strangled its victims, had been brought to heel by the
curative power of antitoxin and, like typhoid, would soon yield to vaccination. In 1905 the U.S. Public Health Service (USPHS) slew the fearsome
dragon of yellow fever, terminating an epidemic in New Orleans by means
of mosquito control. New techniques of contagion control and therapy
diminished the terrors of the great white plague tuberculosis. Paul Ehrlich's "magic bullet" for syphilis, salvarsan, raised hopes that other new
drugs against infectious disease would soon follow. Progressive muckrak-
ers like Upton Sinclair and Harvey Wiley led a fierce crusade to purify the
country's food, drink, and drugs. It was a time of great exploits and public health heroes.[1]

No American exemplified this trend as well as William Crawford Gorgas, conqueror of Panama Canal fevers. This Alabama-born army surgeon
used the discoveries of Ronald Ross and Walter Reed to carry out the
first practical demonstrations of disease eradication via antimosquito campaigns. The Panama Canal had first been a French project, but the ravages
of yellow fever had driven the French from the field in 1889. Gorgas, as
chief sanitary officer of the Panama Canal Commission from 1904 to 1913,
used strict antimosquito measures to make digging the canal a possibility.
His fame in eliminating yellow fever reached so far that it could even become the subject of a madman's ravings in an American comedy published
almost four decades later.[2] Gorgas also attacked malaria, and while he did
not remove it entirely from the Canal Zone, he did reduce the number of
cases by as much as 80 percent. His approach was mainly one of drainage,
screening, use of quinine to treat active cases, and the hand killing of adult
mosquitoes. He enlisted children in this last effort, paying them a certain
amount per dead mosquito harvested.[3]

Gorgas's techniques were labor-and cost-intensive. His budget for malaria and yellow fever control far exceeded the amount of money available
in the southern states for public health work. If southern public health

officials were to have any chance of controlling malaria in the South, they needed to find either a cheaper way to do it or someone else to pay for it. This search dominates the story of malaria control in the South during the first three decades of the twentieth century.

## The Impoverished, Sickly South

By today's standards, the American South of the early twentieth century was a developing country, with weak local governments, a colonial financial infrastructure, and the widespread prevalence of poverty diseases such as hookworm, typhoid, tuberculosis, malnutrition, and malaria.[4] The quandary facing regional public health officials looked very like the hopeless situation faced today in tropical developing countries. The South was, as President Franklin Roosevelt said in 1938, "the Nation's No. 1 economic problem."[5]

Malaria contributed to this poverty. It was a significant source of morbidity for rural, impoverished southerners. Moreover, weak, anemic workers could do little to better their economic condition. Malaria particularly hampered tenant farmers who were trying to keep their families fed by "cropping" cotton, the South's major agricultural product. The fever and chills of *vivax* malaria struck during spring planting season; *falciparum* came along in August and September to keep the worker bedridden on critical harvest days. This reduced economic productivity in turn worsened the sharecropper's poverty, putting quinine, which might have gotten him back out into the fields, beyond the family's reach. People living in such poverty, both black and white, could contribute little to the support of public education, much less public health.[6]

That is not to say that public health activity was absent from the South: yellow fever stimulated extensive local and federal public health work from the 1850s to 1905. Yellow fever is a disease amply endowed with the ability to stimulate public terror and hence generate a public health response. It kills rapidly, horridly, and in great waves, in the process destroying commerce and outraging commercial and political sensibilities. But yellow fever had little lasting effect on public health reform, and once a few years without an epidemic passed, the public health fervor faded away. Fighting yellow fever was not a reliable foundation for stimulating public support of health agencies. And in 1905 yellow fever visited the United States in epidemic form for the last time.[7]

Yellow fever is a disease of towns, ships, and trade, but the main health problems in the South afflicted rural areas. During the first two decades of the twentieth century, the desperately poor health status of rural southerners became a national scandal. The first condition to be exposed was hookworm, a disease in which the parasite passes from fecal material through the skin of the feet and ends up as an adult attached to the lining of the small intestine. Hookworm was rife in the rural South, where both privies and shoes were a luxury. It left its victims weak from loss of blood and nutrients and particularly damaged growing children, badly stunting their physical and intellectual development. This "germ of laziness" made southern workers indifferent and weak, contributing to the cycle of disease and poverty.[8]

The Rockefeller Foundation took up hookworm as a cause in 1909, working for its eradication as a way to create an educated, active workforce. This effort was an expression of scientific philanthropy, as described so succinctly in Andrew Carnegie's *Gospel of Wealth:* the proper philanthropist aimed to avoid charity per se but rather to give the impoverished individual or community the means of promoting their own advancement. Carnegie built schools and libraries; the Rockefeller Foundation likewise targeted education as a means of encouraging economic development, but also promoted medical research and responsible public health. By the latter term they meant public health efforts whose costs fell within the means of the community's coffers, and which local authorities could assume once the demonstration period was over. The hookworm campaign had all these characteristics. It focused heavily on educating people about the infection cycle and urging them to wear shoes and use sanitary privies. In the short term, the hookworm teams also diagnosed and treated hookworm patients in a county fair-type format. In accordance with its philosophy, however, the Rockefeller Foundation pulled out after a couple of years, leaving local officials to wage the battle. Except in Florida, which had an unusually stable public health budget, work on the disease faded with the withdrawal of Rockefeller money.

So although there was some public health activity in the early twentieth-century South, it was limited. Yellow fever was gone, removing a powerful stimulant of public health funding. Hookworm aroused public zeal briefly, then diminished. But awareness of rural illness continued to grow. Pellagra was discovered in the South, where it had no doubt existed for decades or centuries unrecognized. This disease, which is caused by niacin deficiency, is the natural product of a diet consisting of corn, bacon, and molasses. Like hookworm, it causes languor and indifference, making pellagra another "laziness disease" that Joseph Goldberger of the USPHS tied relentlessly to the southern way of life. He mounted a campaign calling for a more nutritious diet as a cure but again ran up against the stone wall of southern poverty and underdevelopment.[9]

The third disease of laziness, malaria, also came to the forefront in the 1910s. It too sapped worker strength and was a major source of rural ill health. But southern public health officials lacked the funding necessary to combat it, just as they could not afford to buy the impoverished southerner shoes or vegetables. Further, the best mode of fighting malaria remained obscure. It was not so much that they did not know how—Gorgas had shown them the way—than that they did not know if there was a method they could afford with the limited public health budget at hand. It was easy, as Joseph Goldberger had discovered, to teach people how to live healthy lives—he had proven at one southern orphanage that he could eradicate pellagra with a nutritious diet. But in the end, that institution had gone back to its initial cornbread and bacon regime, for it could afford nothing better. Likewise, it was easy to tell people to wear shoes and build sanitary privies to prevent hookworm, but it was far harder to pay for them. The public health reformers interested in controlling malaria knew very well that cost was the number-one criterion in making any public health measure acceptable to the politicians voting on the budget.

## How to Do It?

At least four modes of malaria control were available to southerners who were considering a malaria campaign in 1910. There was an ongoing world-wide discussion on the topic, as sanitarians strove to control malaria in Italy, the British colonies of Africa and India, the German colonies of Africa, the Dutch East Indies, the Philippines, and Latin American fruit, rubber, sugar, and rice plantations. The nascent global community of malariologists did not exchange information as rapidly as today via the Internet, but books and journals did flow across oceans at an impressive speed. By 1899, for example, Walter Reed was already very familiar with Ronald Ross's 1897 work. And malariologists the world round were eager to hear of campaign techniques that worked and to share information as well as disagreements.

From the earliest discovery of the mosquito vector and its role in transmitting plasmodia, debate raged about the most effective model for anti-malaria work. One school, championed by Ronald Ross, held that the method was to attack the mosquito at the most vulnerable stage in its life cycle. The larvae floating in pools could be killed by depriving them of water (drainage), smothering them with oil, or poisoning them with toxic compounds such as Paris Green (an arsenic powder first tested in the 1920s). The insecticide pyrethrum was burned in sickrooms to kill mosquitoes, but since its effect lasted only a few hours, it was not a major tool for control. Hand-killing of adult mosquitoes was tried at times, but not until the introduction of DDT to malaria work in 1943 was an effective insecticide for adult mosquitoes at hand. In all these efforts, the focus was on eradicating the mosquito vector, leading at times to the statement that "the mosquito is the cause of malaria" and hence the belief that its death was the ultimate goal.

Proponents of a second alternative put most of their interest into finding ways to kill the parasite in the human body. Robert Koch, among others, preached this gospel. Although he initially proposed using quinine, other agents would be invented and tried as the century progressed. Medications could be used as public health tools against malaria in a variety of ways. The first was to prevent infection (prophylaxis), by taking a pill regularly while in a malarious area. Not until chloroquine was introduced in 1945 was there really an effective medication toward this end. But quinine will reduce symptoms, and so it had some effect. A second use of medication was for "sterilization," or cleansing the parasite from the bloodstream. If it were possible to treat all members of a given community at once and thus eradicate all the parasites, the mosquitoes could bite at will without producing a case of malaria. Overall, the target of this strategy was the plasmodium, not the mosquito.

A third mechanism for malaria control was designed for the European colonies in Africa and was considered in India but was never proposed for the American South. That strategy, described by historian Philip Curtin for Africa, was to separate European "masters" from malarious "peasants" by segregating their housing locations.[10] The European compound would be built at a prescribed distance from the natives' homes, and thus a zone of safety would prevent transmission from malarial carriers to the white colonist. This method was resorted to when quininization seemed not to work and mosquito control was impossible. But segregation never worked very well, partly because total segregation would mean the absence of servants. Further, it aroused the ire of native elites, who refused to be lumped together as "the infected" and who opposed any taxes whose purpose was to better the lives of the Europeans while not improving the lot of the native inhabitants.

Historian John Cell, in a reply to Curtin's paper, has shown that this medically justified segregation lasted only briefly in Africa and never really became established in India at all.[11] Curiously, it never surfaced in the discussions of malaria in the American South, which was at its most segregated in the 1910s and 1920s. But it was embarrassingly obvious that malaria did not limit itself to one race: any segregationist effort would have had to pit class against class rather than white against black, and such strategies never appealed to southern leaders anxious to keep white populism under control.[12] The "malaria free zone" concept did survive, however, in both World War I and World War II, when malariologists at times employed it to describe their efforts to protect sites of military or industrial importance.

A fourth approach to malaria control was to squarely attack the connection between poverty and this disease. Perhaps its most famous proponent was Angelo Celli, who argued that malaria in southern Italy could be alleviated through socialist measures. Although Celli recognized the importance of quinine and protection from mosquitoes, he thought the core of the issue was the poverty of Italy's landless agricultural workers. Social reform was needed to supply the people with nutritious food, adequate housing, and access to physicians and medicine. Alleviate poverty and injustice, he believed, and malaria would recede. A further subdivision of this approach would be to define "adequate housing" as housing with screens to keep out mosquitoes. Although Celli's efforts in Italy were not very long lasting, the question certainly remained active that some component of his plan might work in the American South.[13]

The USPHS became interested in malaria control after the dramatic hookworm campaign of 1909–12. The first step, as with hookworm, was to determine the prevalence of this disease and discover where help was most needed. R. H. von Ezdorf carried out these surveys between 1912 and 1915, documenting the existence of the disease throughout the South. The leaders of two communities—Roanoke Rapids, North Carolina, and Electric Mills, Mississippi—recognizing their economic losses due to malaria, asked the USPHS to organize malaria control projects in their towns. Both were mill towns, with factory supervisors who could easily document the days of work lost to malaria. And both had a lot of malaria—75 percent of the population of Roanoke Rapids had the disease in 1910–13. In both towns the major intervention was to reduce the mosquito presence through drainage. Many people also took quinine, especially after USPHS workers provided extensive educational work about it. The result was a 66 percent reduction in malaria, and great satisfaction on the part of the mill owners about the money they had spent.[14]

The Rockefeller Foundation's International Health Board (IHB) found these initial projects promising. The USPHS did too, but it lacked funds to go beyond what had been done so far. In Roanoke Rapids and Electric Mills, the local mill owners and other civic sources funded the campaigns; the USPHS had very scant resources to devote to malaria work. Wickliffe Rose of the IHB suggested a collaboration: the IHB would fund demonstration projects in selected southern communities, and the USPHS would provide personnel and expertise. The Rockefeller researchers asked two questions: (1) What is the cheapest, most effective method of malaria control? (2) What method is most likely to capture public approval and consequently continued funding? A successful method had to be one that southern towns could afford and maintain after the termination of outside funding. Cooperation with state and local authorities was critical, for in part the projects' purpose was to teach southern public health officials how to manage malaria on their own. The IHB planned to be involved in southern malaria research only for a few years. After discussions among federal, state and local officials, the decision was made to stage the comparative demonstration projects in one of malaria's most hospitable southern locales, the Mississippi Delta. Two methods, mosquito control and parasite eradication, would be tested separately, and the results compared.

During 1916 work began in the delta town of Crossett, Arkansas. The method was simple: control mosquitoes by clearing and improving streams and ditches, and by oiling those bodies of water that could not be cleared or made free flowing. In the first year the IHB/USPHS team obtained a 77 percent reduction in malaria at a cost of $1.24 per capita. In 1917 the town took over the cost, but the Public Health Service continued in an advisory capacity. During the second year, the reduction of malaria was 85.5 percent, at a per capita cost of only $.63. Civic authorities were quite pleased because of the almost complete freedom from mosquito pests.[15] So this demonstration met the IHB criteria: mosquito control was cheap, and popular enough to win local support and funding.

Mosquito control worked fairly well in towns, but towns were not really the most critical malaria sites. In rural areas, widely scattered sharecropper cabins harbored many bodies carrying parasites. Draining and oiling a whole county was just not practicable, since the per capita cost would skyrocket as the area to be drained per person rose. A method of parasite eradication was more appropriate here. The IHB/USPHS researchers wanted to know whether quinine treatment could eradicate the disease, especially in less densely populated areas.

The principal southern figure who argued that quininization could work as a public health measure was Dr. C. C. Bass of New Orleans.[16] While treating patients at Charity Hospital in 1914, Bass had developed a course of therapy that cured them of their symptoms and at the same time "sterilized" the blood of parasites. This regimen, which came to be called the "standard" quinine regimen, was fairly simple. During an acute attack of malaria, for the first few days that the fever and chills prevailed, the patient took 10 grains (650 mg) of quinine sulfate three times a day. Then for the ensuing eight weeks, he or she took 10 grains at bedtime. The idea was first to treat the symptoms and then to "sterilize" the blood by killing all remaining parasites. Hence the first stage of the therapy was of direct and visible benefit to the patient; the eight weeks of daily quinine were intended to prevent a relapse and to eliminate the carrier state, which was of so much risk to the community. Neither rationale for the eight-week course was easy for the patient to appreciate directly. Those people who were loaded with parasites but not clinically ill were prescribed the eight weeks of once-daily quinine alone. This regimen was even harder to market to the individual so stigmatized, because he or she had no direct perception of illness, while the side effects of the quinine (nausea, tinnitus, and headache) were all too obvious. (Dosages were scaled for children, proportional to age.)[17]

In 1916 Bass, along with physicians from the USPHS and the Mississippi State Board of Health, began an IHB demonstration project using such "quinine sterilization" in Bolivar County, Mississippi. They chose Bolivar County because it was as heavily infected as anywhere in the United States. Its population of about 50,000 people, 25 percent white and 75 percent African-American, lived in one of the swampiest regions of the state. After a survey determined that more than half the population had malaria, the researchers handed out free quinine to all who were infected, along with the standard therapy guidelines and instructions on how to follow them. There, and in a later study in Sunflower County, Mississippi, malaria was reduced by 90 percent, at a cost of only about $1.16 a person.[18]

Bass was very proud of his accomplishment. He got the Southern Medical Association and the USPHS to give their stamp of approval to his system of quinine dosage. He also convinced at least one quinine manufacturer to package the pills in the bulk amounts of the standard course of therapy so that the patient would benefit from the reduced cost of larger amounts. Bass became famous as the man who had done so much to solve the malaria problem. But all was not well, as Bass himself knew. The high doses of quinine were good for quickly ending an individual's episode of fever and chills, but on the community level practical barriers to public health success arose. People would not take that much quinine voluntarily—both because of its cost and because of its side effects. Rather, they preferred to take smaller doses for a shorter period of time, controlling both their costs and the side effects of nausea and dizziness. But this abbreviated course might well make them more likely to relapse later (although that could be dealt with in time). Communities were loath to intervene in so personal a transaction as paying for medicines, preferring community drainage projects that fit the familiar model of public works. For all these reasons the standard therapy might work in the experimental setting, but it was not practicable for the long term. Toward the end of his life Bass admitted in retrospect, "The campaign undoubtedly reduced clinical *vivax* malaria, but did little to eradicate it."[19]

Bass continued to promote the standard therapy into the 1920s. He acknowledged that mosquito control might be the better method for cities, but he believed that his plan worked best in rural areas.[20] In 1921 the Mississippi State Board of Health distributed placards promoting the modern use of quinine; in 1922 the USPHS sent out 250 circulars to southern hospitals, proclaiming the worth of the eight-week cure.[21] As late as 1924 a USPHS malariologist was still promoting the efficacy of the standard treatment. His paper followed an Alabama demonstration project using quinine sterilization during 1923, which showed an 80 percent reduction in malarial prevalence.[22] But such projects were becoming more and more rare. Increasingly, when civic or county authorities organized programs to control malaria, they turned to drainage, oiling, and the use of a newly recognized arsenic larvicide, Paris Green. By the end of the decade, few American malariologists, apart perhaps from Bass, felt that malaria could be eradicated in a community by the systematic sterilization of malaria carriers.[23]

Several studies by other malariologists appeared in the mid-1920s that argued against using quinine as a public health measure. In Alabama one USPHS researcher distributed free quinine to malarial households and instructed mothers on the standard course of quinine therapy. After eight weeks, he found, all of those people with previously positive smears now showed no parasites in their bloodstreams. The individuals appeared healthier, felt better, and were more able to work. Yet in the following months, and before the resurgence of springtime mosquitoes, a third of them had relapsed, with evident parasites in their blood. So, he concluded, quinine did not sterilize their blood, even if it did improve their clinical condition and feeling of well-being.[24]

The second influential study was done at Leesburg, Georgia, the site of a malaria research station established by the International Health Board in 1924. There two field malariologists chose 74 black children with splenic enlargement, a prominent sign of malaria in children. One-third of the children went into an untreated control group, and the rest received the standard therapy, although for twelve weeks instead of eight. In 1925 the researchers experimented with lower doses of quinine in half of their treatment group and higher doses in the other half. They discovered that quinine cleared the blood of parasites, and that the spleens began to recede. But when the quinine was discontinued, the spleen grew again and the parasites returned. So they concluded that quinine had little use as a public health measure. Comments following the presentation of this paper at the Southern Medical Association meeting in 1925 showed that quinine sterilization had become a touchy and controversial subject. Several physicians chimed in that their own research corroborated the findings. But others were upset that the standard treatment was under attack. "[T]he Virginia State Board of Health has thoroughly advertised the value of the standard treatment," one Virginia official moaned. If the board had to reverse itself now, "we would in large measure lose the confidence of those upon whom we must rely to help us carry out our malaria control program. From an administrative standpoint, at least, such a course would be disastrous."[25] Still, it was hard to argue with the continual flow of studies showing the inefficacy of quinine as a public health measure. Another International Health Board–funded malaria project in Brazil supported the rising swell against quinine as a control agent, finding that the expense involved was not worth the cost of the intervention.[26]

One of the principal reasons that quinine therapy declined as a public health measure is that it so depended on the cooperation of individual patients and doctors. As H. R. Carter said in 1920, quinine prophylaxis "is best suited for a community either very biddable or very intelligent and well instructed." He went on to add, "In the South I would take my chance with the country negroes as being the first rather than with the white farmers as being the second."[27] Other health officers struggled to get their people even to accept the mosquito vector theory, much less to buy into the eight weeks of quinine therapy. In describing one Virginia education campaign in 1922, the state's health officer despaired at the population's ignorance, stubbornness, and fatalism. "They are told that mosquitoes are responsible for malaria. . . . They are told that watermelons and fodder and muscadines and chinquapins and 'night air' and decaying vegetation and going in the 'old swimmin' hole' on Sundays are not the cause of malaria."[28] Another commentator pointed out that his population needed a lot of help in discriminating between "Divine providence and devilish mosquitoes," for it was both fatalistic and suspicious of new ideas.[29]

By the early 1930s malariologists were expressing pessimism that any drug or combination of drugs was of use as a public health measure. W. E. Deeks, who directed malaria control for the United Fruit Company (UFC) in the Caribbean and Central America, rejected the possibility emphatically. "Mosquitoes can be infected when fed on malaria carriers who are taking full doses of quinine. That question has been solved beyond doubt," he commented at the Southern Medical Association meeting of 1929. "Apparently no amount of quinine will prevent mosquito infection. Neither will it prevent infection in man." He agreed that 15 grains a day would keep a man at work in the tropics, but as soon as he came home to the United States and stopped the therapy, up popped the fever. Deeks went on to admit that plasmochin, a drug that came into use in the late 1920s, did kill gametocytes (the parasite stage picked up by mosquitoes). Physicians on UFC plantations had tried a combination of quinine and plasmochin, the first to treat symptoms and the second to sterilize carriers, but the experiment failed. Initial studies of plasmochin had begun in 1926, but toxic reactions were frequent, and a few deaths even occurred. Reduced doses were then tried, and they did appear to clear the blood of gametocytes. But the real endpoint—decrease in the malaria rates—did not follow. Only mosquito control measures—drainage, larvicides, screening—had reduced the amount of malaria, from 240 to 80 per 1,000.[30] Another commentator said he had gotten better results from plasmochin, but he admitted that its usefulness was limited by its side effects, including a tendency to turn the recipient's lips blue.[31]

Lewis Hackett, the Rockefeller Foundation researcher who was one of the most influential malariologists of his generation, summarized this pessimism about medications for malaria control in his landmark study, *Malaria in Europe,* first published in 1937. While he praised quinine for its effect of interrupting the acute attack of malaria, he saw it as capable of preventing neither infection nor transmission. Atabrine, a drug synthesized by Germans chemists after World War I, had similar efficacy to quinine but higher toxicity in children. He dismissed plasmochin as costly, toxic, and ineffective. Hackett's book presented mosquito control as the only feasible method of malaria limitation, and every malariologist in the United States soon became familiar with his arguments.[32]

Other American voices agreed with this appraisal. W. V. King, chairman of the National Malaria Committee and entomologist for the Department of Agriculture, concluded in a 1938 review article on the history of malaria control that the therapeutic method—medications—had been abandoned. King remarked that "the method was not now a hopeful one, being difficult to apply successfully or economically," and that "[t]his appears to be the majority opinion among malariologists at the present time." King believed rather that with proper knowledge of the behavior of anopheles species in the American South, control would ultimately come from attacking the juvenile mosquito.[33] After more than ten years of research on the subject, researchers at the Gorgas Memorial Laboratory in Panama likewise dismissed the value of medications.[34] This research appeared to settle the question. Atabrine would be given to American troops during World War II in order to prevent the clinical cases of malaria that would debilitate their fighting strength, but all acknowledged that it was a stopgap measure. At least up to 1945 and the introduction of chloroquine, the Kochian plan of malaria control via parasite destruction had failed.

The third option for malaria control, that of creating malaria-free zones, did have some success, but it really functioned as a subset of other methods. The concept of separating the carriers of malaria from the uninfected, as suggested in Africa or India, could not be applied in the United States. Carriers could not be easily distinguished by race, so any such segregation would have depended on the laborious and expensive task of checking blood samples, which was simply impracticable. Malariologists did retain the concept of the zone, however, and applied it along with mosquito control. In World War I and again in World War II, circles of protection were drawn around sites of military importance, such as training camps and significant industrial installations. Military sanitarians took care of the area in the circle within their jurisdiction; various local, state, and federal authorities completed the job. So the zone concept did persist, along with the notion that it was more important to protect some people and places from malaria than others.

The fourth option, Celli's concept of social reform as a measure against malaria, was never seriously considered in the United States. Even in the New Deal of the 1930s, the idea of handing out a straightforward dole to alleviate poverty was short-lived. But one aspect of socioeconomic improvement was explored by the Rockefeller researchers and implemented after the great Mississippi River flood of 1927. The housing of the southern rural poor was so pathetically inadequate, and particularly so porous to mosquitoes, that it seemed worthwhile to invest in improved housing to see if this would reduce the malaria prevalence. Because early studies had demonstrated that malaria control could be easily and cheaply accomplished in towns through environmental measures, the housing studies focused entirely on the problem of rural malaria. In towns drainage needs were limited and could be paid for by a relatively large tax base. But to free only one or two rural houses from malaria, the same amount of drainage work might be necessary as was needed for a whole town. So the question was framed: which worked better, a quinine program or a screening program? As we have seen, quinine did not work. As with the initial quinine studies, the research on housing improvement was done on the poorest of the South's poor, the tenant farmers of the Mississippi Delta.

The principal crop of the Delta was cotton, a product that was well known for making a few large landowners wealthy and creating an underclass in desperate poverty. Certainly these folk, who were 80 percent African-American, lived under dismal conditions. One survey found that the average occupancy per cabin, both black and white, was 6.1 people, all crammed into two or three rooms. Cash was short, and the tenants paid in cotton for their privilege of living in the cabin, using the landlord's tools, and purchasing essentials before the crop came in. This was a highly mobile population, as families moved from plantation to plantation, trying to improve their lot. But the poor quality of housing from landlord to landlord varied lit.tle.

The houses were notoriously bad. The roofs leaked, there were gaps in the walls, and children worried about snakes coming up through the holes in the floor. A wood- or coal-burning stove, which provided heat for warmth and cooking, was vented through an open chimney. To retard rotting of the floorboards, cabins were usually built up on blocks, which provided an ideal daytime retreat for mosquitoes in the dark caverns underneath. The landlord had little incentive to improve the housing stock, and the frequently migrant workers treated the shacks with contempt. Cabins were often located in clusters, on the least arable land of the plantation. While the plantation owners chose their own building sites that had advantages of elevation, breezes, and distance from mosquito breeding grounds, the sharecropper cabin frequently bordered swampy land. Although *de jure* segregation to prevent malaria from infecting the "master race" was never explicitly practiced in the South, in actuality the location of housing accomplished much the same result.

As part of the Rockefeller demonstration projects in 1916–17, Lake Village, Arkansas, was chosen as a site to test screening of such houses as the sole intervention. Public health workers fanned out over the demonstration area, screening houses and repairing other gaps in the cabin infrastructure to make them as mosquito-proof as possible. This effort was accompanied by an educational project. Tenants were taught not to kick a gap in the screen door by using a foot to close it, to protect the screens on windows from similar damage, and to paint the screens once a year to keep them rust-free. Further, they tried to convince the tenants to sit inside the screened areas in the early evening, rather than on the cooler open porch. By and large, the tenants were initially cooperative and appreciative. The first year the project brought in impressive results: a 70 percent reduction in malaria, at a cost of $1.75 per capita. In the first year of follow-up the screens remained in good order, but a later survey found them increasingly neglected. The major reason was worker mobility, as after a few years the cabins' occupants were not the tenants instructed in the first year of the project. Screening was not a "once and for all" matter but required ongoing maintenance and education.[35]

Two audiences were taught the gospel of screening. One was the landlord who owned the cabins; the other was the tenant who had day-to-day contact with the screens. Malaria workers ultimately deemed both audiences obstinate and ignorant.[36] Planters typically believed that their tenants could not and would not take care of property, tools, and livestock, and they saw little purpose to wasting money on any sort of improvements.[37] The tenants could be just as difficult to convince, although some authors noted that black tenants were more compliant than white. One USPHS physician told a typical anecdote about a white tenant farmer, whom he described as moving from farm to farm every year or two: "I asked him if he did not think it was important to screen his house. He said 'Yes.' He could not 'lay down' and take a nap in the summer time without being troubled by flies." The patient official tried to build from that knowledge to an understanding of malaria. "I suggested that would be one reason, and I said malaria would be another. I said you get it by the bite of the mosquito. He said, 'I have heard that.'" The physician's exasperation broke through when the man admitted, "'I did have malaria in about five places I have been, and I did lose one child at the last farm I lived on before I moved here.' That is how seriously they consider the malaria problem. He thought he had lost that child by some other means. He did not think he was responsible."[38] As another public health official put it, "We can reconstruct houses, but how far can we go in reconstruction of habits and impulses that are characteristics of the class under consideration?"[39]

A more serious barrier to screening was that many sharecropper cabins simply could not be mosquito-proofed. A USPHS physician writing on "rural malaria control" in North Carolina raised just this dilemma. "But what of the Negro tenant 'shack'?" he asked. "Totally unscreenable, often built within easy-flight range of an extensive swamp or marsh, and in a highly malarious neighborhood. It would seem that these were beyond the pale and outside the scope of the worker in malaria control."[40] The issue was not the application of screens to shanty windows and doors but the overall porosity of the construction, so that mosquitoes had multiple sites of entry. One solution was to cover the wall and floors with kraft paper, the kind of heavy brown paper from which grocery sacks are made. But kraft paper was even less likely to last than the rustable screens and was hardly practicable in a house full of children. The obvious solution was to build new houses, with screened porches and tight construction. Designs for such houses were published in the public health literature. Some organizations made a point of following the patterns, such as TVA, which built worker villages with screened houses at new construction sites. But in the long run, as a permanent public health measure designed to help the majority of the rural southern poor, screening worked no better than quinine.

At the heart of the problem was tenants' lack of power over the landlord, who determined the quality of housing stock available. Occasional organized screen promotions, such as the screening campaigns at Lake Village, Arkansas, a 1930s push to screen cabins in the swampy riverside counties of western Tennessee, or the screens provided throughout the Mississippi Delta by the Red Cross after the 1927 flood, were only temporary measures. As late as 1939, one Arkansas tenant told an interviewer, "We misses screens de mos' aroun' dis place, pesky flies and mosquitoes is so bad. I said sump'n about it to Mr. Roper early dis spring, but I guess he forgot— or mebbe he ain' forgot, he jus' doan' *want* us to have no screens."[41] Ultimately, the landlord had to be convinced that minimal standards of housing were necessary for the health and efficiency of workers.

Out of these various forays into malaria control, a consensus emerged. Although screens and medication had their place, the cheapest, most reliable, and ultimately most practicable mode of malaria control was to attack the mosquito, whether in its larval form or as an adult. This was feasible in towns, where drainage programs created new land for construction, and a more affluent population appreciated the comforts of screened houses and a life with fewer mosquitoes. Given the available tax base in towns and cities, urban areas soon significantly reduced and even eradicated malaria during the 1920s. But rural areas had the most stubborn portion of the South's malaria cases. In these areas, there simply was not enough money in county or state budgets to meet the overwhelming costs of antimosquito work, and quinine had not worked. Deeper pockets were clearly needed. Large industrial and agricultural enterprises offered one potential source of such largesse.

## Selling Malaria Control

When approaching the middle and upper classes about malaria, public health officials strove to convince them that having malaria cost more than preventing it. While researching my first book, on the history of yellow fever and southern public health, I found that business interests played a surprisingly large role in combating epidemic disease. The reason yellow fever was so powerful a stimulant of federal, state, and local public health efforts was principally that it sapped trade, not that it had a major impact on mortality figures. Yellow fever was a destroyer of commerce, and commercial men responded to its depredations. In regard to malaria as well, the opinions and actions of southern businessmen bear importantly on the story. As in the case of yellow fever, reformers, in arguing for measures against the disease, were aware of the influence that the affluent could bring to bear on government spending and thus emphasized the financial consequences of malaria. The economic argument worked well for some groups, such as the railroad, lumber, textile, and hydroelectric interests, but it mostly failed to penetrate the managerial minds running the South's plantations.

Using a term sure to stir up the affluent, malariologists warned that a "malaria tax" was automatically being added to the cost of goods produced, since ill workers were inefficient workers. In 1913 a group of public health reformers used such an appeal in seeking money from the Rockefeller Foundation for antimalaria work in the South. Echoing the justification that had worked so well for hookworm, their proposal proclaimed that malaria "leaves its subjects anemic and neurotic and is responsible for inertia, loss of will power, intemperance and general mental and moral degradation. It is probably the greatest foe to the development and progress of the South." Like hookworm, malaria was a germ of the laziness that blocked the South's economic development. The proposal went on to describe the costs of malaria in more detail. "The economic loss, aside from the deaths it occasions, is wrought (a) to the individual through loss of time, money expended, and diminished efficiency (b) to the community through reduction of real estate values, difficulty of inducing immigration," and so on. The committee claimed that malaria led to $100 million a year lost due to disease.[42]

Many employers bought this argument, especially ones who contracted to provide medical care for their workers. In 1914 the owners of cotton and paper mills in several towns invited the USPHS (in the person of Henry Rose Carter) to study their communities' malaria problem, which kept so many of their workers idle. Frequent worker illness reduced productivity since skilled workers could not be instantly replaced, and production plans had to be curtailed due to absences. Carter studied the problem and made recommendations, which the mill owners funded. Their gratitude shines through the USPHS reports on the projects, which doubled as demonstration sites for other mills. One mill manager "stated that at no time has labor been more efficient and sufficient, attendance more steady, and sickness less, and that the returns for the contribution of $1000 of this one mill were more than gained in one month's . . . operation." Another mill manager glowed, "The money spent in antimalarial work here has paid the quickest and most enormous dividends I have ever seen from any investment, and after having had our experience I would, if necessary, do the work over again if I knew it would cost ten times the amount."[43] The Roanoke Rapids project, and a similar one that followed in the lumber mill town of Electric Mills, Mississippi, became models for showing the economic benefits of carrying out antimalaria work in the mill village. Other mill managers and owners were quickly won over with this data.

Railroad managers were also easily impressed. Railroad lines ran through some of the most malarious regions of the South; think of the romantic *City of New Orleans* going past the houses, farms, and fields of the Mississippi Delta on its regular run from New Orleans to Memphis to Chicago. Both the Illinois Central (owner of the *City of New Orleans*) and the St. Louis Southwestern Railway Company transported cotton and lumber out of malarious areas and depended for their prosperity on the health of their own workers and those out in the fields and woods. Railroad management had led discussions on the need to reduce yellow fever in the late nineteenth century, so it was accustomed to equating health with wealth and development. The Cotton Belt Railway, a subsidiary of the St. Louis Southwestern line, first began antimalaria work in 1917. The chairman of the board of directors, Edwin Gould, had been disturbed by how much time his workers spent in the company-supplied hospital being treated for malaria. He set up a private fund to explore and implement ways to reduce this amount of disability. The company borrowed J. A. LePrince and T.H.D. Griffitts from the USPHS and had them make a survey and recommendations. It then hired a full-time sanitary engineer, H. W. Van Hovenberg, to supervise the work.[44]

Van Hovenberg quickly realized that protecting the railroad's own workers was not enough. If the industries that supplied goods for the railroad to carry were working less than efficiently because of malaria, then the railroad suffered in turn. So his measures tended to be widely inclusive of the towns through which the trains passed, and he worked to gain the cooperation of local and state authorities as well as local business owners. "Since the cost of labor is the greatest expense in maintaining railroads, there should be, and there is, a direct relation between the cost of railway maintenance and the malarial index of the country through which the railroads operate," he wrote in 1920. "The railroads can justify their financial support of malaria work in cities and towns through having a more efficient labor supply to draw on, through protection of employes [sic] and their families, and through the increased prosperity of the towns."[45] The town of Lufkin, he said, was an example of a community where local interests worked with the railroad to control malaria. In Lufkin the railroad paid five-ninths of the cost, and the Lufkin Land and Lumber Company, along with a local philanthropist, made up the rest. At Keltys, Texas, the San Augustine Lumber Company paid the entire cost of the malaria control efforts, while the railroad engineer helped with planning and implementation. In both cases the communities were able to ship about 20 percent more lumber (via the railroad of course), and the investment paid for itself.[46]

The voices of railroad magnates spoke loudly in Texas, and Dallas financiers listened. One spokesman for the Dallas Chamber of Commerce explained the connection: "As a business proposition we have learned in Dallas, Texas, the biggest inland cotton market of the world, that we cannot grow cotton on Main Street, not does it thrive among our towering skyscrapers." Businessmen therefore had to pay attention, he said, to the status of cotton growers in east Texas who produced the crop marketed through Dallas. They had to be "interest[ed] in malaria control for purely commercial reasons." Accordingly, as the representative of the Dallas Chamber to the East Texas Chamber of Commerce, he joined in sponsoring a bill "appropriating $50,000 for the specific purpose of malaria control and empowering the State Department of Health and the United States Public Health Service to launch such a campaign." He also helped organize a letter-writing campaign to the governor and state legislators. "The difference between $50,000 for control work and $50,000,000 for neglect was so obvious that letters from no less than 200 of the outstanding business and professional men of the State were filed with the Legislature." He had no doubt that "they were the balance of power that secured the money."[47] Although public health writers frequently argued that the case for malaria control should be put to men in power in just such language, it is unusual to see it so lucidly laid out and played out.

Other public health lobbyists had similar luck with economic arguments. An Alabama strategist believed that it was key to show a profit of at least $1.50 for every $1.00 spent. "We had one community last year in which we made a house-to-house canvass twice during the year. The figures given by the people show that in 1919 they spent for doctors, quinin [sic], chill tonics and loss of wages, $26,245," he reported. "We did some malaria control work in 1920 costing $3000.00. That year malaria cost them (again according to their own figures) $521.00. In other words, they saved $25,724 on an investment of $3000—a return of over 700 per cent." Using these figures, the state board of health convinced many other communities to take up malaria work.[48] Another malariologist working for the USPHS in New Orleans agreed: "In the matter of appropriations, legislatures can best be influenced by facts and figures that show the dividends to be derived."[49]

Planters were much harder to reach than the merchant class. Southern public health officials were repeatedly stymied in their attempts to influence this group. "The land owners in areas with malaria tell you either they have no malaria in their community or they do not care if they have," said one official from Montgomery, Alabama. "If the tenants become sick, they will get others."[50] A USPHS engineer commented similarly on the difficulty of convincing planters that malaria control was in their best interest. "Plantation farming can be likened to a specialized form of industrial establishment. The cost of operating the plantation is made up among other things of fertilizer, seeds, implements, mules, and labor," he reasoned. "Labor, however, is approximately 50 per cent of the production cost. We find the plantation owner studying methods, best use of implements, rotation of crops, markets, so forth. Why does he refuse to become interested in the one item that is 50 percent of the total cost of production, labor?"[51] In one western Tennessee campaign to put screens on sharecroppers' houses, the state paid for part of the cost, organized the production of cheap screens for windows and doors, and ran an educational campaign. The landowners had to make only a fairly small contribution, and most joined in. However, "[o]ne large land owner gave us to understand that she would never do any screening," reported one article on the project. "We screened all around her property, and when tenants began to move to other places where mosquito proofing was available, she changed her mind. Of course her house was screened."[52] The argument that more efficient workers created greater prosperity penetrated slowly into the planter class.

Much of this slowness was due to denial—"We have no malaria here." F. J. Underwood, the head of the Mississippi State Board of Health, ran into this problem repeatedly. He claimed that during 1924 the loss from malarial fever in his state amounted to more than $2 million. In order to quantify the economic difference that malaria control could make, he compared two counties in which the malaria prevalence was known due to state surveys: one had malaria control and one did not. He wrote the chambers of commerce in both towns and inquired how much cotton had been harvested by the end of October, "requesting information as to the reason for the amount so far taken out of the fields." In the county with malaria control, 75 percent of the crop was in, and the report praised two factors: the weather and the health of the labor force. "The Secretary of the other Chamber of Commerce reported the crop to be about 45 per cent gathered, giving the reason that the shortage of labor had proved a great handicap." Yet he also said that malaria "had interfered very little with cotton picking, according to information received from the planters themselves." Since the counties were similar with regard to weather, soil quality and so on, Underwood concluded that the critical difference in productivity was due to malaria, even if the planters refused to see what was right under their noses.[53]

It is difficult to know how often planters were persuaded by economic arguments, since the evidence is largely anecdotal. A few years after the Underwood comments cited above, another public health official made some headway with a group of Mississippi planters. He credited educational work done by the American Red Cross after the 1927 flood with having some impact on the planter perspective. "We were then in a position to approach the planter about the work. We showed him the cost of sickness, loss of time, doctor's bills and funeral expenses." After explaining how much malaria was costing him, the official went on to detail the costs of malaria work. "We proved to him that it costs very little more to screen a home, which was a permanent protection for three or four years from flies as well as mosquitoes, day and night, than to furnish mosquito netting for the beds which last only one season." What really convinced this group, however, was the plan to bill the costs to the tenants themselves, with payback due with the fall crop. But the usual response was indifference. Even when presented with data like that collected on one large Mississippi plantation in 1915, which showed more than a thousand worker days lost to malaria during the cotton-growing and -harvesting seasons, or that the impact of malaria amounted to a tax of $3.88 an acre, the planters did little without subsidy from outside agencies.[54]

## Hydroelectric Malaria

In terms of commerce and industry, malaria had its most significant impact on the development of hydroelectric power in the South. Although waterpower had been developed as early as the late eighteenth century in New England, it was not until around 1900 that developers seriously began considering harnessing the South's streams to make power. Between 1900 and 1930 dams went up all over the southern piedmont. Duke Power Company, founded in 1905, had ten hydroelectric plants in North Carolina and South Carolina by 1925, growing side by side with the booming textile industry. Multiple other power companies, including most prominently Alabama Power Company, built dams on southern rivers big and small, so that by 1930 the plants were generating five billion kilowatt-hours annually, providing electricity for homes and industry over more than 120,000 square miles of the South.[55]

All of this power came with a price, however. Whenever companies dammed a river to capture the water's "white coal," they also created a lake behind the dam, where water once flowed. The miles of shoreline increased with the area of pond, and since anopheles most like to breed on pond edges (and not in running water), the opportunities for mosquito propagation escalated geometrically. Another problem was that the reservoirs were sometimes not cleared in advance: some companies just flooded the valley behind the dam without doing any sort of preparation, submerging all the trees, other plants, and existing structures in the process. Gradually they would break up into rotting parts and float to the surface. As one USPHS malariologist said of such an unprepared reservoir, the river "left in its backwater, trees, brush, logs and flotage—the Anopheles' idea of 'home beautiful.'"[56] If even one case of malaria existed in the area for the resulting hordes of mosquitoes to feed on, the result was a malaria epidemic.

As with yellow fever and quarantine, public health officials were in a quandary as to how to protect vital commercial interests as well as the health of the people. Henry Rose Carter, the USPHS malariologist who first studied the issue, recognized that "[the] problem was a large as well as an important one." Since "on it, to some extent, depended whether the water power in the malarial sections of the United States could be developed economically," it became critical to find ways to prevent the "damage which its development would cause the health."[57] Every writer on malaria and the impounding of water (as the creation of a pond or reservoir by building a dam was called) recognized that "the health authorities' duties are . . . two-fold—protection of the public health and assistance in a tremendously important, legitimate industrial development."[58] The South desperately needed the economic development that cheap electric power would bring; hence the investors in such companies were not dissuaded by or even very interested in outbreaks of malaria.

Who had the power to tell hydroelectric power companies that they had to pay attention to malaria? Because they made use of a public resource, navigable rivers, there was considerable legal precedent for oversight by federal and state governments. The first time Congress addressed the issue of hydroelectric power was in 1884, when it allowed a project only under the supervision of the Army Corps of Engineers. Multiple other individual acts followed, each one considered on a case-by-case approach. During World War I the federal government went into the hydroelectric power plant business when President Wilson authorized construction of a dam on the Tennessee River at Muscle Shoals, Alabama, to be located close to two plants for making explosives. Although the project was unfinished at war's end, it had set a precedent and became the nucleus for the Tennessee Valley Authority, which would be created in 1933.[59]

Most projects in the first three decades of the twentieth century were instituted by private companies, however, which had to deal variously with the Department of Agriculture, the Department of the Interior, and the secretary of war in understanding federal requirements. These requirements could be contradictory, at the whim of individual government officials. In 1920 Congress created the Federal Power Commission to bring these interests into one office, which was given the authority to regulate 85 percent of the country's potential waterpower streams. The commission established procedures for obtaining leases and licenses, set standards for dam construction, and helped ensure the safety of investors' money by providing professional supervision. The government was not yet in the business of generating or selling hydroelectric power, but it had established its right to regulate it.[60]

By 1920 much was known, from experience with actual outbreaks, about the relationship of impounded water to malaria epidemics. As a result, the power companies more easily accepted the regulatory actions of the Federal Power Commission. There had been scattered malaria problems around impounded water in 1910 and 1912, but the 1914 outbreak along the banks of the Coosa River in Alabama laid the track that all other hydroelectric power projects would follow. In 1914 the Alabama Power Company closed Lock 12 of the Coosa River, creating a large artificial lake in a basin that had received no prior preparation. What followed was "the greatest outbreak of malaria that the State had ever seen."[61] The community responded by filing multiple damage suits against the company. The company settled out of court, promising to clean the pond's edges properly to reduce the malaria problem.[62] Henry Rose Carter and his colleagues in the USPHS, J. A. LePrince and T.H.D. Griffitts, made a detailed study of the Coosa River and other cases and arrived at a series of provisional recommendations for companies to follow when impounding water.

The key goals were twofold: to keep the malaria parasite out of an area, and to avoid providing the mosquito with an ideal breeding ground. Excluding the parasite particularly meant screening imported workers for malaria and treating all those infected with quinine. Conducting a malaria survey of the district beforehand was also useful, for two reasons: infected residents could be treated, which would decrease the likelihood of a subsequent outbreak, and the power company could document that malaria had existed in the place before the new pond was formed, which could provide a handy defense postimpoundment if a family brought suit for the creation of malaria. The second goal, preventing mosquito breeding grounds, involved clearing the potential reservoir. The company sold the lumber and had it cut and hauled away; the remaining brush was cleared and burned. As much as possible, the sides of the reservoir were cleared of overhanging trees and bushes that could add debris to the shores of the pond. Once the reservoir was formed, aquatic plants likewise had to be cleared. If these efforts proved unavailing in preventing larval breeding, then the water could be sprayed with oil or Paris Green. Finally, Carter and others showed that rapid fluctuation of the reservoir water level would strand the larvae and flotage on the shore, or drown the larvae with lapping waves.[63]

These methods all cost money, of course, and the power companies were not in business for anyone's health. Two forces acted to bring them into compliance. The first were regulations, issued by the Federal Power Commission (after consultation with the USPHS) in 1922, that made it impossible to get a federal license without agreeing to follow the antimalaria rules.[64] Several states passed similar regulations, with Alabama in the lead in 1923. The laws were tested by the River Falls Power Company, which began building a dam on the Conecuh River near Gantt, Alabama, in 1922. After doing some clearing and promising to follow the regulations, the company proceeded to flood the reservoir before it had been properly prepared. A severe outbreak of malaria followed. The state board of health issued recommendations to ameliorate the situation, but the company ignored them. The state's attorney general then took the power company to court. As S.W. Welch, the state's chief public health official, reported in 1927, "We did not give in one inch, and at about the time the trial was to come up they said they were willing to obey the regulations."[65]

A second and probably more powerful force driving the power companies to cooperate with public health agencies was the threat of lawsuits. The Coosa River case established the precedent. A similar scenario was played out near Decatur, Georgia, where a dam was built in the early 1920s by a company that completely ignored the state's suggestions (not yet regulations) about preparing the reservoir and conducting the work so as to avoid malaria. "Late in the summer of 1926 certain citizens living near the pond entered suit for damages against the company," reported the state's health officer at a meeting of the Southern Medical Association that year. "Before the date of trial, a meeting of the attorneys and health officials was arranged, and the power company agreed" to a variety of antimalarial measures suggested by the state.[66] Likewise, when the construction of a dam near Louisville, Kentucky, was followed by a malaria outbreak, "they had a tremendous amount of litigation," according to the state's health officer. "Lawyers and doctors were kept busy giving expert testimony on both sides, and it was a lucrative business for them, and disastrous for the power company."[67]

Caught between the devil and the deep blue sea, the power companies found it cheaper in the long run to abide by the regulations. Then if malaria did flare, they could argue that they had done everything necessary to protect the populace and that the epidemic was the result of an "act of God," not negligence on their part. A Georgia public health official commented in 1929, "The cooperation now being received by the State Board of Health from the various power companies is very gratifying." He was pleased to report that "the time has arrived when power companies value the control of impounded areas not only as an important health measure, but as a legal protection to the power companies."[68] A spokesman for Duke Power Company expressed the same point of view even more graphically. The former custom of creating a reservoir with no regard for public health, he pointed out, had led to malaria and several hundred thousand dollars in lawsuits. "If a company wants to get down and out, let public sentiment turn against it. When it has a batch of law suits it will go down rapidly," he lectured. "Most companies realize this and in the past few years have made every effort to keep their ponds clean and in sanitary condition and see that the laborers who are used in the developments are protected against malaria."[69]

The Duke representative went on to praise the protection offered by a good preimpoundment malaria survey: "Our general attorney called at my office last spring and asked me about certain people living in this area who were talking about bringing suit for malaria against the company. I looked back in my records. In this family of seven five gave a history of malaria two years before the impounding project. . . . All I had to do was to give this to the lawyer and when he told their attorney they had had malaria previously he knew it was useless to bring suit."[70] Among lawyers, bringing such suits had become something of a cottage industry. By the late 1920s the companies had generally become so compliant, and the lawsuits such a nuisance, that public health officials were more likely to praise the power companies and condemn the litigators than the reverse. "Here we have a condition where business executives are carrying on . . . malaria control operations on a much larger financial scale than all other anti-malarial activity in our country taken as a whole," acknowledged one malariologist who was later to work for the TVA. "Those who are doing the best sanitary work are being attacked and robbed for doing applied sanitation. . . . [T]hey are frequently subject to legal attacks."[71]

It is hard to know whom to have more pity for, the power companies or the plaintiffs. The other point of view was represented poignantly by a poor Alabama woman in 1938. (The dialect is from the original interview.) "Ain't none of us much healthy," she began. "Ever' since th' power company backed this river up mor'n twenty year ago, they's been chills an' fever hyar. It ain't bad as it was right atter they built th' dam, but it'll still kill you." Then she told a story about a neighbor's fight against the power company.

> It ain't funny to be sick, but they's funny things happen. When they first built th' dam, Ol' Man Mac come down with chills so

hard that he shuk th' bed posts, an' he liked to died. . . .[W]hen
he got outa bed, th' first thing he done was to go hell bent fer
. . . a lawyer . . . an' sued th' power company fer th' biggest
figger of money he could think of. Well, that lawyer had a slick
tongue. He had Ol' Mac thinkin' that th' money was as good as
his already, an' they wasn't nothin' left to do but cash th' check.
That ol' man went looney crazy. He run aroun' tellin' people he
was go'nter be rich, an' he bought up as much as he could on a-
credit. . . . 'Course he didn't git nothin'. . . . He might a
knowed that they ain't no pore man can win nothin' off'n th'
power company.

She did acknowledge, after telling this sad tale, that she and her neighbors
were illegally squatting on the land, which limited their rights to sue for
damages. "That's the trouble tryin' to live on a river," she said, "'specially
a river that's full of backwater. Since the power company built that dam,
there's been sickness up and down these banks all the time. But can't anybody lay blame on the power company. They own this land we're livin' on,
and they didn't ask us to come down here in the first place." Still, she was
bitter at the way the power company had treated her people. "They look
at us folks hyar on th' river like we'uns was no better'n a dog. A pore man
don' stand no more chanct than a June bug in January."[72]

From reading the medical literature, one would conclude that by 1930
all the power companies accepted the need to clear reservoirs and otherwise protect against malaria. This woman's narrative tells a different tale,
but it is difficult to judge the typicality of her experience. The TVA certainly took the malaria lesson to heart and, by the end of the 1930s, became
one of the principal actors in malaria control. Yet the same story of poor
preparation and explosive malaria was repeated with the hasty impoundment of water behind South Carolina's Santee-Cooper Reservoir in the
1940s. The power companies in general became strong advocates of preventing malaria through proper engineering, but when the restraints of
regulation and litigation were lifted in the war fever of the 1940s, it was all
too easy to slip back into negligence toward the public's health, especially
when that public was poor, black, and rural.

## Three Decades of Experience

By 1930 public health officials in the South had learned much about controlling malaria. It was a fairly easy disease to control in towns, and by
drainage and other antilarval methods, urban cases had become rare. Funding of urban projects was not difficult, since local governments were easily
impressed by the monetary argument for mosquito suppression, as well as
the popularity of mosquito reduction among voters. The "man-made"

malaria that followed the construction of railroads or the impounding of water was largely under control, as management came to understand the financial tax that raging malaria imposed. Indeed, even on the southern cotton plantations malaria was subdued, although it was not by any means gone. Significant progress seemed to have been made, thanks to the tools of modern science and the wisdom of southern civic and business leaders. The events of the next decade would shatter such complacency.

# Chapter 5

# "A Ditch in Time Saves Quinine?"

The Great Depression decade was a pivotal period in the history of American malaria. While the first half of the 1930s saw a massive surge in malaria cases, the disease had almost disappeared by 1940. These years offer fertile material for a historical analysis of the causes of malaria's progress and retreat. It was a time of major socioeconomic turmoil, and the decade saw the implementation of federal relief efforts on a scale never before attempted in the United States. And malaria never recovered from the nadir reached by 1940. During the last quarter of the 1930s, something irrevocable happened to banish the disease.

In 1930, the South remained desperately diseased and impoverished, and its public health apparatus was accordingly underfunded. Malaria had declined over the 1920s, but it was still a visible and troubling presence, and hope was slim that internal monetary resources would appear to aid in its control. There was broad agreement that malaria drained the economy of productive workers. There was equally broad agreement that the South's taxpayers could not afford to pay for the massive effort that would be needed to eradicate malaria from the rural South using the available methods. Even if legislators had been willing, the burden of other diseases (pellagra, hookworm, tuberculosis, and syphilis) hardly made malaria special enough for particular attention, and the pervasiveness of poverty meant that precious few tax dollars were available to spend. Cotton culture bred a wretchedly poor worker class that in turn occupied shabby housing in the swampy countryside. How could change, and increased health, be brought to this system? Or as one reporter concluded, after surveying health conditions in the impoverished rural South in the 1920s, "The solutions to the problems of malaria and hookworm are quite clear—draining, screening, furnishing shoes to the people, and teaching them cleanly habits." But could it be done? Actually, he concluded, "the whole thing is as simple and easy as it would be for a one-armed man to empty the Great Lakes with a spoon."[1]

## Malaria in the 1930s

As in the third world countries that the South of this era resembled, aid had to come from the outside, in the form of charitable contributions or governmental interventions. We have seen the role that the Rockefeller Foundation played in some of the earliest antimalaria campaigns. The USPHS was also active, to the extent that its funding allowed. The Rockefeller Foundation eventually pulled out, deciding to target international health problems instead. The USPHS saw its budget cut by the penurious Coolidge administration in the 1920s, then lowered still further by the early years of the Great Depression. Other philanthropic agencies, who would otherwise have been willing to continue their work in the South, had to withdraw as their investment income crashed along with the stock market in 1929. As desperate poverty settled over the South in the 1930s, malaria made a dramatic comeback, reaching incidence levels not seen since 1912.

Surprised public health officials had not expected the spike. By the early 1930s the prevalence of malaria in southern "urban" areas (population greater than 1,000) had declined markedly, thanks to drainage and larvicidal efforts, and it appeared to be declining in rural areas as well. Although not subject to the dust storms of the prairie states, the southern region did experience drought, with a resulting drop in the anopheles population. Consequently, the years 1930-32 marked a new low in malaria mortality rates. Malariologists at the state and national level began to sound rather smug. As a Georgia public health official summarized, "We have passed through a dark period . . . and at times our problems seemed almost hopeless. We are now emerging from this period and feel very optimistic."[2] They had the disease on the run and felt that it was only a matter of time before it was gone altogether. "[M]alaria in Mississippi is slowly becoming a vanishing disease," claimed statistician Frederick L. Hoffman in 1932. The future indeed looked bright, although the era's economic desperation prevented total equanimity.[3]

Imagine the dismay when the malaria mortality rate soared in 1934 and 1935.[4] This resurgence destroyed all hopes that the disease would gradually fade away, for it had come back with a vengeance. Tulane epidemiologist Ernest Carroll Faust kept track of malaria mortality data, gathering, publishing, and analyzing each state's reports yearly. In 1945 he presented a cumulated version of his results, beginning with 1929.[5] Information about disease-specific mortality before that year was incomplete, as not all southern states participated in collection and reporting. Faust's table indicates that malaria mortality rates generally declined up to 1932, peaked from 1933 to 1936, and gradually dropped thereafter.

Mortality data as a source of information on malaria has its problems, given the poor quality of reporting and the large margin of error between

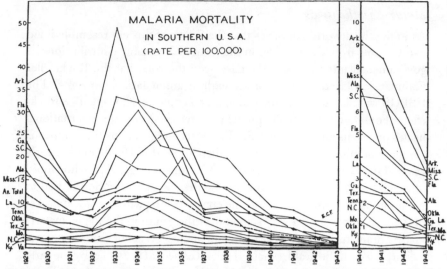

Fig. 1. Chart showing the year-by-year malaria mortality rate per 100,000 population for each of the fourteen malarious states in the southern United States, 1929–1943, together with the average rate each year for these states. On the right the rate scale is enlarged for the years 1940–1943 for the purpose of clarification.

Malaria Mortality in Southern U.S.A., 1929–1943. Ernest Carroll
Faust of Tulane University gathered U.S. malaria mortality statistics
each year and in 1945 published this cumulative graph. Malaria
peaked after the Mississippi River flood of 1927 and again during
the depths of the Depression, while it so declined in the 1940s that
Faust had to alter the scale to reveal the details.
("Clinical and Public Health Aspects of Malaria in the United
States from a Historical Perspective," *Am J Trop Med* 25 [1945]:
185–201, at 191)

counting deaths and counting cases. Most states made no attempt to collect accurate morbidity data until the 1940s; that is, they did not ask doctors to report cases of malaria along with the patient's name and the result of a blood film examination. The only records available for most of the twentieth century are mortality reports, which means cases of malaria that ended in death. Such mortality data is limited in many ways. In the first place, most people who get malaria do not die from it, so these cases are not counted at all in mortality lists. If every death from malaria were recorded accurately, one would have to multiply the mortality rate by anywhere from 200 to 400 to approximate the actual number of malaria cases. Mortality data was flawed for other reasons as well. Often the cause of death was arrived at only after the person had died, based on the reporting of family members or the opinion of the county registrar. Doctors' premortem diagnoses were not routinely on record. Many southerners never saw a doctor, choosing instead to self-medicate with chill tonics or herbal concoctions; others viewed the chills and fever as so much a part of life as not even to be classified as illness.[6]

Nor did a medical degree ensure that a diagnosis would be accurate. Southern physicians were prone to calling all fevers, malaises, myalgias, and headaches "malaria" and to treating them with quinine.[7] One epidemiologist summarized, "A case of malaria is a rather indefinite something which the best authorities have not been able to define for precise statistical purposes."[8] Physicians tended to use quinine as a diagnostic aid, concluding that if a fever went away with its use or the person otherwise got better, then the cause of infection was malaria. Since many viral infections, for example, will resolve spontaneously, this method left a lot to be desired as a diagnostic test. A physician might also be reluctant to report the true cause of illness. Some insurance policies that paid death benefits specifically excluded certain diagnoses, such as tuberculosis or syphilis, so malaria might make a handy substitute. Or the actual disease might be shameful in some other way. My father contracted murine typhus in 1944, when he was working at the local farmers' co-op. Murine typhus is carried by rats and their fleas, both of which are common around feed supply stores. He got over it, after a period of hospitalization, but as far as the world knew, he was suffering from a bout of malaria, not something as dirty and shameful as typhus.[9]

A diagnosis not only had to be made accurately, it had to be reported properly if it were to enter the historical record. Busy physicians were often reluctant to abide by state laws that required the reporting of cases. A 1939 parasite survey of an eastern North Carolina county found 392 positive smears; 40 percent of those patients had seen a doctor and been told they had malaria, but none of the cases had been reported to the state board of health, as required by law.[10] In other instances, to satisfy the law, physicians made a rough estimate of the number of malaria cases in their practice. In the late 1940s, physicians were required to supply actual patient names, as opposed to a conglomerate number, at which point malaria cases dropped dramatically. Still, the morbidity and mortality data from the twentieth-century South is all that is available, and it probably gives at least a crude idea of the malaria parasite's presence and distribution.

Official death statistics are not our only window into malaria's changing prevalence in the 1930s. More accurate, but more limited in scale, were malaria parasite surveys done by public health investigators in communities. During such studies, field-workers gathered drops of blood from the survey population to be examined for parasites, and recorded information about disease symptoms, doctor visits, treatment, and socioeconomic status. Data from such studies suggests that malaria had decreased even more markedly during the late 1930s than Faust's graph would suggest. Blood surveys during the mid-1930s commonly showed parasite rates of 5 to 10 percent, and a typical estimate of total southern malaria morbidity based on such rates was five million cases.[11] One Tennessee Valley Authority malariologist commented in 1946 that while he and his colleagues had discovered only twenty positive smears in their northern Alabama surveys of 1943 (or 0.13 percent), they had usually found that many cases in two or three houses alone in 1934. Particularly unfortunate communities had rates of 50 to 60 percent positive smears in that year.[12]

Other studies support this rapid drop in malaria rates between the mid-1930s and the early 1940s. For example, the North Carolina Board of Health routinely surveyed children from 1937 to 1945, in the malarious eastern counties. Whereas in the late 1930s the board's surveyors commonly discovered average rates of 5.5 percent infected in some schools, and even 62 percent infected in one county, by 1943 they could find only 17 positive slides for every 10,000 children tested.[13] The cumulative figures for slides examined from all the southern states were similar, with a 0.3 percent parasite rate in 1942 and 0.09 percent for 1943.[14] One USPHS disease tracking station, set up in a Georgia county notorious for malaria, found no positive smears after 1944 and so had to convert its primary research focus to mosquitoes instead.[15] So two things need to be explained: why did malaria escalate in the mid-1930s, and why did it just as rapidly disappear by the early years of the next decade?

The reasons for the escalation appear to be grounded in the sudden worsening of the already severe state of southern poverty during the Great Depression. As discussed earlier, poverty spurs malaria in multiple ways. Although quinine is not effective as a malaria eradication tool, it does suppress the disease and enable the person taking it to perform work; but hard times put its purchase out of reach for many. Quinine does reduce mortality and also may decrease the likelihood of gametocyte production, lessening the transfer of disease. If the Rockefeller studies did not find malaria eradication with quinine use, they often found significant malaria suppression. In fact, in those studies, with the discontinuation of quinine, malaria bounded back, which is the pattern seen in the 1930s. Shutdowns in industry moved population out of the "urban" areas, where jobs had disappeared, and back to the country, where at least a little sustenance could be scratched from the land. Although mosquitoes had been significantly controlled in towns, little had been done in the countryside, so that such migration to rural areas increased the likelihood of anopheles bites. Agricultural production waned as tobacco and cotton prices bottomed out, and land previously drained and plowed lay fallow, growing puddles and breeding mosquitoes. As one public health official put it, "While many farms have gone out of cultivation almost every available house in the country is now occupied by some family (often undernourished) which has returned to the land while attempting to weather the depression." Poverty bred malnutrition, reducing the immunity that had previously kept malaria in check in many southern bodies.[16]

It is fairly easy to propose reasons that malaria got so much worse in the mid-1930s—one expects hard times to breed disease. But what happened toward the end of the 1930s and in the early 1940s to erase this peak in incidence? The rest of this chapter will attempt to answer this question, with a principal focus on the infusion of federal money into the South. New Deal programs did have a decided impact on the banishment of malaria, but hardly in ways that could have been predicted as the decade opened.

### The Works Progress Administration

The early 1930s were a time of severe contraction of public health budgets, especially for southern boards of health that were long used to operating on the most threadworn of shoestrings. Malaria control efforts mostly just stopped for lack of continuing funds. The U.S. Public Health Service budget shrank markedly, and its support for malaria projects likewise faded. Public philanthropies such as the Rockefeller Foundation and the Rosenwald fund were unable to pick up the slack. In the face of mounting malaria cases, public health officials had none of their familiar supports for mounting a new effort against the disease.[17]

Help actually came from an unexpected quarter. After Franklin Roosevelt took office in March 1933, his administration inaugurated the first of a series of New Deal programs to alleviate unemployment that were also to become central to malaria control. In the spring of 1933 the Federal Emergency Relief Administration (FERA) began doling out relief payments nationwide and, in a small way, approached the task of putting men back to work. Several southern state boards of health took immediate advantage of this program by employing these relief workers in drainage projects.

Any able-bodied man could dig a ditch, they reasoned, and the more swamps drained, the less malaria. "A ditch in time saves quinine" became their motto, and this simple adage guided almost all of the malaria work done in the United States during the mid-1930s.[18] When the Civil Works Administration followed in the fall of 1933, the Public Health Service submitted plans for malaria drainage as a project worthy of manpower expenditure. Over the next four months, an average of 64,000 workers were busy digging 6,000 miles of ditches, which drained more than 300,000 acres of wetlands.[19]

In 1935 Roosevelt responded to the critics of FERA by ending the direct federal dole and pouring money into a new agency, the Works Progress Administration (WPA). Its specific task was to pay men and women to work in the community, at a rate above that of welfare payments but below the usual wage for such work. By 1936 the WPA reported on 735 projects in 29 states, including the famous Writers' Project, theatrical productions, and construction projects erecting schools, hospitals and other public buildings. But these projects all required skilled labor. Work was needed for the unskilled unemployed, and it was such tasks that earned the WPA the nickname "the shovel brigade."[20] Some of these shovels were wielded in the creation of new roads and sewers, but a significant proportion of the unskilled WPA laborers in the South were digging ditches to drain swampland. Over 36,000 men worked on WPA malaria projects in the spring of 1936, draining three million acres at a cost of more than $15 million.[21] The Social Security Act of 1936 included emergency funds for the U.S. Public Health Service, and these were added to the budget for drainage.[22] Most of the drainage work was done by the end of 1936, and afterward in the wake of the conservative attack on the New Deal, funding for the WPA dropped.

It is difficult to evaluate the quality of this federal program. Because the work was so poorly planned, the records that could help in this evaluation, such as high-quality morbidity outcome data, do not exist. This was not because professional knowledge of how to organize and measure such a campaign was lacking. For example, E. L. Bishop, the state commissioner of health for Tennessee, clearly outlined the way a malaria project should be orchestrated in 1933. First the areas of malaria's prevalence should be determined, preferably by blood smear screening of children in the fall (for *falciparum*) and in the spring (for *vivax*). Then the area should be topographically mapped, and the sites of anopheles breeding identified. Only then could the sanitary engineer know which wetlands most needed drainage. The next step was to design a drainage system that actually did drain the wet area and did not worsen the problem by creating new standing pools. Finally, arrangements needed to be made to maintain the drainage ditches. A dirt ditch will quickly silt up and become clogged by leaves, sticks, and other debris. Instead of facilitating drainage, it will host new anopheles populations. Maintenance of the ditches was a critical part of the work, one that demanded long-term commitment from the community.[23] Then the effect of the project could be measured by follow-up surveys.

How close did the New Deal public works projects come to following this ideal scenario? Not very. As one *Southern Medical Journal* editor summarized in 1933, "[T]he rapid and unexpected manner in which . . . funds were made available has resulted in execution of some ill advised or poorly executed drainage."[24] Another evaluator commented later, in 1939, that since WPA funds had been used without expert supervision, "the work has proceeded in such a way that the neglect of a few years will duplicate the conditions remedied."[25] Men had to be employed immediately, so there was no time for the recommended fall and spring surveys.[26] There were not enough engineers to help guide the work, so instead state boards of health rushed to issue at least basic guidelines on ditch construction.[27]

There is ample evidence that contemporary malariologists frequently found the drainage work wanting. Suggestively, the one investigator who tried to gauge the effectiveness of drainage programs by comparing drained and undrained sections of his Mississippi county in 1936 found no difference in the malaria rates.[28] Another documented that malaria had increased in some counties in 1935, in spite of miles of drainage ditches.[29] By 1938 multiple authors reported that the malaria rate was steady or increasing, despite all the money spent on it.[30] One army medical man noted in that year that "the very general prevalence of the disease fills many with a feeling of hopelessness" because the problem seems "insoluble on account of the area involved and the great cost of preventive measures." He went on to predict that "it is not possible that within the lifetime of the present generation any state in the endemic area can become practically malaria free."[31]

This is not to say that the drainage programs had no effect at all. Certainly they had their fans. Surgeon General Thomas Parran claimed in 1938 that the WPA drainage effort had advanced U.S. malaria control by twenty years.[32] A WPA publication claimed that "a tremendous advance in the control of malaria has been made in recent years. . . . Under these . . . programs almost 2,000,000 acres of swamps have been drained, affecting the health of 15,000,000 people."[33] In North Carolina, for example, by February 15, 1937, 922 miles of ditches had drained more than 12,000 malaria-breeding acres. "This malaria control program, which already has given unmistakable evidence of its immense help in combating one of the most stubborn diseases," was, according to a letter from the state health officer to the state WPA administrator, "of vast importance to the thousands of people who live in the areas where these projects have been underway." Yet far from eradicating or reducing malaria, even he had to acknowledge that there had been a "general increase in malaria."[34]

In part, the statistics may be misleading precisely because the intervention brought men into the vicinity of the anopheles in great numbers. Workers hired to dig drainage ditches have to work next to the swamp being drained and thus have greater exposure to mosquitoes and to any parasite carrier among the work crews. So it is possible that malaria rates first rose in response to this stimulus, then fell again when the drainage reduced anopheline populations. Nowhere have I found data that is fine enough to reveal this sort of detail. Nor does the sort of tracking exist to help us follow a tract of land over several years to see if it persisted in a dry state, and hence remained anopheles-free, after the WPA crews left. No doubt some of the drainage helped reduce malaria in some places, but I have not found the expected large drop that a program that involved such impressive acreage and money would imply.

Adding to the difficulty in judging the effectiveness of the drainage program was the tendency of the Republican opposition to characterize many of the New Deal projects as "boondoggles." The Memphis WPA office was lambasted, for example, for building a $25,000 doghouse, when it fact the money had been spent for a rabies control plan that included a new dog pound.[35] H. L. Mencken spoke for this side when he criticized the waste and foolishness of the WPA efforts in 1936: "Instead of safeguarding the hard-earned money of the people . . . , [Roosevelt] has thrown away billions to no useful end or purpose." Mencken was particularly harsh in describing the WPA managers as "blatant and intolerable idiots," a bunch of "quarreling crackpots, each bent only upon prospering his own brand of quackery and augmenting his own power."[36] In the light of such overt political causticity, it is hard to know whom to trust on the question of the competence of WPA managers. Still, it is hard to find spokesmen in praise of the WPA malaria work who were not somehow directly involved in producing it or benefiting from its funds.

One circumstance that lessened the impact of the malaria control projects was the way they were distributed across a state's geography. Malaria might be located only in the coastal or river valley counties of a state, for example, but all the counties needed and received relief money. Thus a large amount of "malaria control work" was done in counties with only the vaguest suggestion of malaria's presence. The details reported in the Tennessee Department of Health's *Biennial Report* for 1933–35 were typical of accounts by southern state health officials during this period. Table 5 of that report lists county-by-county information on miles of new ditches dug, miles of old ditches cleaned, and the number and area of ponds and swamps drained. The document then goes on to present a map of counties doing malaria work. Most of the malaria in Tennessee during the 1930s occurred in the two-county-wide band of lowlands bordering the Mississippi River. But as this map shows, "malaria control" projects were happening in many other counties where malaria prevalence was minimal indeed. WPA funds and employment relief was first on the minds of government officials managing these projects, not the most efficient ways in which to spend money for malaria control.[37]

In fact, the point of the program was never really malaria control but the creation of jobs. A public health official excused the shoddy work done in Arkansas with the caveat, "[I]t is realized that the primary purpose of these projects is to aid in unemployment."[38] A Tennessee reporter echoed this view, noting that although most funds for public health had been cut, the "labor project" of digging ditches went forward.[39] No attempt was ever made to figure out *where* drainage would be most effective for *malaria control*, and one explanation of why the money spent had little impact on malaria rates is that the "malaria lands" were among the least likely to gain attention.

The quality of the work was also questionable. Most of those thousands of miles of ditches were simple dirt troughs, and they quickly became silted up, allowing the land to reaccumulate water and revert to its prior situation. Rarely did the work meet the specifications defined by one engineer in 1940: "Malaria control drainage is a very specialized type of work and should not be undertaken unless well qualified, experienced engineers are available to select, plan, and supervise the work." Otherwise, "the whole investment . . . [will have] been lost."[40] Work was planned so poorly that one malariologist later said of such projects, "Too often in the past, drainage ditches have been dug up hill, so to speak, by workers with no knowledge of engineering practices. Likewise, ditch digging specialists have drained areas of little or no importance in malaria control."[41] The speed of the program's onset did not allow for the few available sanitary or civil engineers to consult on projects. Laypersons planned most of the ditches, with predictable results. There may have been areas where WPA workers made a significant local impact on malaria rates through well-constructed permanent drainage systems, but little evidence indicates that the programs significantly changed the malaria prevalence rates over the long term.

## The Tennessee Valley Authority

The history of the Tennessee Valley Authority, on the other hand, is a saga of heroic deeds well done, which really did bring untold benefits to the people while preserving their health. The idea for the TVA came from Senator George Norris of Nebraska, who had argued from the mid-1920s that one governing body should be in charge of the Tennessee River's enormous potential for hydroelectric power. The concept grew out of the controversy over what to do with Wilson Dam, which the army had built on the Tennessee River during World War I. Various private groups offered to buy it from the government, including one headed by Henry Ford. Norris suggested instead that it be the first of a chain of such dams on the Tennessee River, run by a federal agency that could bring flood control, erosion prevention, and cheap electric power to the Tennessee valley. His suggestion fell on deaf ears as long as Presidents Coolidge and Hoover were in power, but he had better luck with Franklin Roosevelt. On May 18, 1933, Roosevelt signed the bill creating the TVA. By 1936 there were plans for nine high dams on the Tennessee and its tributaries, with Norris and Wheeler Dams actively under way.[42]

It did not take long for the TVA to recognize its particular responsibility with regard to malaria. Its malaria control program began in northern Alabama, in the vicinity of Wilson and Wheeler Dams in 1935. A department of health and safety was created in that year, with Eugene Bishop, for the previous ten years the state health officer for Tennessee, at its head. From the beginning the emphasis was on cooperation—cooperation with the Alabama and Tennessee state boards of health, with the USPHS, with consultants from the Rockefeller Foundation, and with entomologists from the Department of Agriculture. One malariologist even spoke of the "TVA model" of malaria control, by which he meant the merger of various experts, such as medical malariologist, sanitary engineer, and entomologist, into one working team.[43] Furthermore, the various goals of the TVA were pursued in harmony. "It can be stated that there should be no conflict whatsoever between hydro-electric development and health conservation," said one TVA engineer. "Rather the two are workers together for the common good; water power promoting industrial and social progress, and public health providing an atmosphere in which enterprise can live and move."[44]

Not everyone loved the TVA, of course. It endured three years of court challenges from 1936 to 1939, spearheaded by those who feared socialism was creeping insidiously into the heartland. There was much anguish and loss as the reservoirs created by the dammed Tennessee River flooded former homes and communities. Ultimately, the power generated by the dams, and the recreational opportunities created by the reservoirs, would bring an economic rejuvenation to the region, thus becoming one of the main engines of southern sunbelt prosperity. Even in the short run, in the dark days of the mid-1930s, it took a lot of labor to build those dams, and each man's paycheck sent a ripple effect through his community where it was spent on food, clothing, medical care, and other necessities.[45]

Bishop, head of the health and safety division, from the beginning focused not only on active antimalarial measures but also on malaria research. Scientists funded by the TVA, both men and women, studied many projects related to malaria. These included: the behavior and life cycle of *Anopheles quadrimaculatus,* epidemics in the reservoir areas, techniques for dusting large bodies of water with Paris Green and later DDT, effectiveness of herbicides in clearing aquatic vegetation, and methods of water level fluctuation in relation to larval breeding.[46] Aside from the vast research effort launched against malaria during World War II, the TVA funded more malaria research than any other institution in the country, and its scientists produced first-class work. The impoundment of the Tennessee River could have generated malaria rates not seen since the nineteenth century; it is vastly to Bishop and company's credit that this did not happen.

The control of malaria on the reservoirs was itself an ongoing experiment, as methods were tried, results evaluated, and systems refined. The reservoirs were cleared with great care before impoundment, and side tributaries were filled to eliminate peripheral standing water. Where larvae bred in spite of reservoir preparation and water level fluctuation, teams went out in boats to spray the larvicide Paris Green or oil on the lake edges to kill the larvae. My mother remembers the oily beaches on Watts Bar Lake during World War II, particularly since she was under stern orders to keep the dog from rolling in the greasy mess.[47] TVA engineers experimented with spraying Paris Green from airplanes, and in the mid-1940s they would spray DDT in the same way, testing it as a larvicide.[48] When the Kentucky Dam and reservoir joined the TVA system in 1944, the TVA workers took additional steps to avoid a malaria outbreak, going so far as to mosquito-proof houses within one mile of the lake and to distribute pyrethrum to the households.[49]

As with all measures taken deliberately against malaria, it is difficult to judge the efficacy of the TVA effort. The area of northern Alabama where the first TVA malariologists worked had previously been highly malarious, but by 1944 malaria was no longer there.[50] Some of this reduction was due to the effect of the Wilson and Wheeler Dams themselves, as the sluggish tributaries and overflow ponds that flanked the Tennessee River were submerged under the reservoir. Since *Anopheles quadrimaculatus* breeds on the edges of lakes, and those edges were kept clean by the TVA, the dams likely had the double effect of eliminating prior breeding sites and not creating new ones. Otherwise, we are left with that great conundrum of public health and preventive medicine: if the disease does not come, can we take credit for preventing it? Would it have come if we had not intervened? Where there are control populations in similar circumstances, without intervention, then comparison is possible. But such pristine experimental conditions existed nowhere in the American South, least of all in the TVA region.

The WPA projects may have created malaria in some areas and reduced it in others, but they probably had little overall impact on malaria morbidity and mortality. The TVA definitely controlled the disease in areas under its jurisdiction, but they were limited, after all, to the Tennessee River valley. The TVA also made a major contribution to malariology via its support of research into malaria control, in an era when the U.S. government had limited funds for field epidemiology. A third federally funded intervention in the South actually, albeit inadvertently, increased malaria.

## The Santee-Cooper Power Project

In 1941 dams closed on the Santee and Cooper Rivers in South Carolina, generating much-needed power and causing an explosion in malaria cases. Malaria had been a severe problem in the South Carolina low country ever since the first African slaves imported *falciparum* malaria in their bodies to the swampy region near the Carolina coast. The area surrounding this new hydroelectric installation had a smoldering reserve of malaria cases that caught fire when hordes of mosquitoes bred on the reservoirs created by the project.

The Santee-Cooper project has been described as a "little TVA," and in many ways it fits that description. After their efforts in the 1930s had failed due to lack of capital, backers of a hydroelectric power plant on the Santee-Cooper system succeeded in acquiring federal support for the program. The $31 million that the project required was 2.5 times the state budget of South Carolina in 1939; no one but the federal government could have come up with so much money. Almost half the money was given as an outright grant, the rest as a federally guaranteed loan. Included in the plan was the use of WPA laborers, who did much of the unskilled work of clearing land and excavating soil. Contract lumber companies took the trees that were commercially valuable; WPA workers then cleared the rest of the land by burning the residue. Nine hundred families left the land, and the power authority built them new houses nearby. All together it took only two and a half years to clear 171,000 acres of swamp and forest, move 42 million cubic yards of dirt, and pour three million cubic yards of concrete.[51]

One engine fueling this rapid pace was the demand of wartime industries for power. The power plant was designated "necessary for national defense" by the National Defense Board in early 1941, and the rate of construction increased as a result. One casualty of this acceleration was the clearing of the upper reservoir. The consequences of poor reservoir preparation had been amply demonstrated earlier in the century, when surfaces of newly impounded bodies of water provided ideal environments for mosquito propagation. Without sufficient clearing, a lake surface would be coated with debris where mosquito larvae could hide from their natural predators, top-feeding minnows. A clean bottom and shoreline, on the other hand, left the larvae without cover. This fact was recognized by state and power industry alike by the early 1920s, and lawsuits brought by the victims of malaria outbreaks around new reservoirs made the alternative of proper initial clearing economically viable. Accordingly, there had been no malaria epidemic fueled by newly impounded water since the 1920s. The TVA research of the 1930s offered excellent guidelines for water impoundment. But in the case of the Santee Reservoir, many trees were still standing when its waters covered them over, and the shoreline was also uncleared in many spots. The decision to proceed regardless was deliberately made by the project's public health consultants in order to speed completion, for the need for power was increasingly urgent. So as the dams closed, the waters filled an only partially cleared Santee valley. "This is why, even today," noted the official historian of the project, "Lake Marion [the upper, Santee Reservoir] has a wild, untamed appearance as compared with to the more placid look of Lake Moultrie [the lower reservoir]."[52]

Not surprisingly, the project generated mosquitoes and hence malaria. The Public Service Authority and South Carolina State Board of Health were aware of the phenomenon, and in early 1944 they prepared a report summarizing the malaria problem and asking the USPHS for help in controlling the disease. The USPHS then prepared an intensive survey of the area, including the epidemiological, entomological, and engineering features of the reservoirs and a rim of territory surrounding them. It found that the lower Pinopolis Reservoir (later Lake Moultrie) had been well cleared and now produced only small malaria hazard. The Santee Reservoir (aka Lake Marion) was a different kettle of fish. Under its surface lay more than 47,000 acres of dead trees, with a consequent dense flotage of logs and other debris on its surface. As the initial sanitary report on the reservoir summarized, "Much heavy standing timber is therefore present in the central part of the reservoir. This is largely dead or dying and causes huge piles of log jams, drifting logs and small debris."[53] There was also an abundant growth of aquatic plants such as alligator grass, whose herbaceous meshwork created refuges for mosquito larvae escaping hungry top minnows. This vast water surface offered ideal breeding conditions for mosquitoes. Accordingly, the Santee Reservoir produced an abundant crop of anopheles mosquitoes in that summer of 1944.[54]

The USPHS researchers visited as many homes as they could in the area within 1.5 miles of the reservoirs, taking blood from every willing inhabitant. They sought people at work in the cotton fields, resting at home, or attending school, and they stuck a finger of each one. The blood slides were then sent to a USPHS laboratory in Memphis, where the results were subsequently punched onto IBM cards. The project ultimately coded almost four thousand names.[55] On the north shore of the Santee Reservoir, 39 percent of the population had visible parasites in their blood. Another area just below the Santee Dam showed around 15 percent positive. Adjacent to these regions, around 8 percent of those tested were proven infected, while the remaining areas (especially around the lower reservoir) were lightly affected. *Falciparum* was the principal species of parasite, although some *malariae* organisms were found. Almost all of the residents were African-American, so *vivax* was rare. It was not unusual for everyone in a family to be infected, and some houses held ten to fourteen people. Mosquito surveys found a correspondingly densely infected anopheles population.[56] The federal response to this burst of malaria was part of the DDT campaign that will be explored in Chapter 7. The Santee-Cooper area was one of the first domestic testing grounds for DDT spraying, and then later in the 1940s became part of the overall Communicable Disease Center initiative to eradicate malaria throughout the South.

The DDT program did not begin until 1945, yet malaria was almost gone from the South (except around the Santee-Cooper Reservoir) by 1942 or 1943. What caused this diminution? The WPA programs to control malaria were ineffectual; the TVA helped eradicate malaria in limited areas; and the Santee-Cooper project actually generated malaria. The programs that directly targeted malaria thus cannot be credited with the overall disappearance of malaria from the South. As it turns out, one federal initiative with no malaria ambitions at all, directed at the economics of southern agriculture, probably had the biggest impact on malaria prevalence—and that as an unintended side effect.

### Location, Location, Location

Before turning to this significant federal intervention, it is worth reviewing the factors most important to the perpetuation of malaria. As noted earlier, diet, access to medical care, adequate housing, the presence of livestock, and the concurrence of other diseases all play roles in the prevalence of malaria. But the most important factor in the history of American malaria, I believe, is the proximity of people to mosquitoes. Relocation was arguably the principal means by which settlers in the Old Northwest rid themselves of malaria—they moved away from the riverbanks and drained the land surrounding their dwellings. The anopheles mosquito usually does not venture more than a mile from its watery birthplace. When people move out of that radius, the chain of malaria transmission, fragile in the American subtropics, is easily broken.

In my research on malaria, I had hoped to find the sort of detailed data set that would let me pass judgment on the relative importance of different aspects of the parasite's biography. But the quality of malaria morbidity and mortality data is so poor, even for the 1940s, that a detailed analysis based on, say, general mortality reports and census data would be so flawed that its results would be of little value. The very localness of malaria makes even county-level data inadequate for the sort of fine correlation that could help determine which socioeconomic and geographic factors were most important in malaria's generation. Still, I was fortunate to stumble over a small collection of malaria surveys that offer some insight into these larger questions.

In 1938 and 1940 the North Carolina State Board of Health conducted town malaria surveys in the counties of its "malaria belt" in the eastern lowlands, bordering the coast. With the exception of communities that lie right on the beaches and harbors, eastern Carolina remains today a region of swamps and rural poverty, and some communities are composed almost entirely of African-Americans. Most of the material gathered in surveys was published in summary form only. It was my great good fortune that the current North Carolina state medical entomologist, Dr. Barry Engber, called my attention to some rotting records that he had found in a barn that had been used for pesticide storage. Many of the yellowed pages were moldy or rat-chewed beyond use, but a few packets remained intact. The records had two components. The first was a set of town maps, with all of the houses numbered and the geographic details, such as lakes, roads, and railroads, drawn in. The second was a series of notebooks with the following survey information for each house:

1. Names and ages of occupants
2. Race
3. Whether the house was owned or leased
4. The quality of the house, ranked from A (best) to E (in need of major repairs)
5. Which occupants had malaria last year (by family report, and if possible, by doctor's diagnosis)
6. In families with malaria, whether they called a doctor or self-medicated
7. Number of the house, which correlated with the maps

This information allowed me to look at the relationships among race, class (using house type as a proxy), and geographic location *vis à vis* the likelihood of having a case of malaria in the house.

Some interesting information resulted. Blacks and whites called doctors at about the same rate; one suspects that levels of poverty were not that far apart for whites and blacks, with the exception of the few obvious landowners who always had a doctor. Whites had malaria more than blacks in the various communities surveyed, which is to be expected this far north, where *vivax* malaria was more common than *falciparum*.

Most significantly, prosperity, as measured by house rating, seems to have been less important a factor than proximity to town pond. Of the few complete data sets I have for eastern North Carolina, most villages were so dominated by ponds that the number of houses out of the anopheles flight range were insufficient to make for a good comparison with those within flight range. But the village of Bowden, in Duplin County, provides a useful test case, for a fair proportion of its houses lay more than a mile from the town pond. Bowden, an agricultural community clustered around Bowden Lake and lying alongside a railroad track, had 120 households in 1940. The 205 people with malaria were just as likely to live in quality houses as in the worse shanties (although admittedly the majority—five-sixths—of the houses were in poor shape). In other words, socioeconomic status does not predict malaria in this little town. But proximity to the pond does. People living within a mile of Bowden Pond were 11.5 times as likely to get malaria as the people living outside that one-mile radius. Location mattered more than money, at least in this case.[57]

How generalizable are these data? Not surprisingly, it is hard to say for certain. In other instances of malaria outbreak mapping, such as around the Santee-Cooper Reservoir in 1945 or the Gantt Reservoir in Alabama in 1925, the risk of getting malaria is clearly correlated to proximity to the water source and its disease-carrying anopheles.[58] Another data set comes from Oliver Wendell Holmes, whose 1834 report on malaria in Massachusetts maps a similar localized outbreak—again, one mile around a new mill pond.[59] The differential impacts of geography and poverty are difficult to tease out, since the affluent always tend to choose to live higher and drier than the poor. But in the case of the southern sharecropper, the location of their cabins on the least arable, most boggy land made all the difference in their exposure to anopheles mosquito. Any set of events that caused them to move elsewhere should have caused a corresponding depression in malaria rates, especially since by the end of the 1920s, malaria was controlled in larger southern towns and cities. Moreover, since *Anopheles quadrimaculatus* bites mainly from dusk to early morning, the person's location during those hours matters most. So even if a farm laborer worked in the cotton fields all day, if he lived in town at night, his malaria risk was lowered.

## The Agricultural Adjustment Act

The federal program that most reduced malaria in the American South during the 1930s was one that promoted rural depopulation and thus moved malaria carriers and potential malaria victims away from mosquito breeding grounds. In 1933 Congress passed the Agricultural Adjustment Act (AAA), which paid farmers to take their land out of cotton, tobacco, and rice production and provided investment capital for the purchase of machinery. This act affected the malaria rate in two important ways. Since fallow land is more likely to develop drainage problems and breed malaria, its first impact was actually to increase malaria cases. But more important, a rural depopulation followed from the act, since to landowners the incentives for capital investment and decreased land use made large-scale farming more profitable than renting out small parcels to tenants.[60] Landlords demolished tenant cabins in order to use the land they sat on, ended sharecropping agreements, and hired the former tenant farmers back as day laborers. Sometimes they had to use violence to force the laborers off the land, and in an Arkansas case tenant farmers tried to fight this process through collective action. The rural shack dwellers moved to town, or to the north, losing in the process their close proximity to the swamps.[61]

The impact of the AAA on the South was nothing short of dramatic. In the late 1930s and early 1940s, Gunnar Myrdal, whose sociological analysis of race in America—and unabashed attack on southern racism—was published in 1944, directly witnessed the depopulation of the rural countryside. "Few Northerners have any idea that the Negroes are being pushed off the land in the South," he wrote with anger. He blamed this process on the development of world cotton competition, as well as "a *national* agricultural policy discriminating severely against the Negroes." The result fundamentally reshaped southern society. "The Negro has left his seclusion. A much smaller portion of the Negro people of today lives in the static, rather inarticulate folk society of the old plantation economy." "This mass movement of Negroes from farms to cities and from the South to the North," he noted, "has, contrary to expectation, kept up in bad times as in good, and is likely to continue."[62] Ironically, this federal program to boost the agricultural economy, which instead generally made the rich richer and the poor poorer, had a side effect of nearly eradicating a poverty disease. The federal money, which first paid for tractors and later supported the acquisition of mechanical cotton pickers, erased forever the social niche of the southern sharecropper.

This outmigration from the southern countryside contributed significantly to breaking the chain of malaria transmission. Historian Jack Kirby has written that during the late 1930s the "southern countryside was . . . enclosed and depopulated as dramatically as rural England toward the end of the 18th century."[63] After the Civil War, black southerners had already begun to move north and west, a migration that accelerated in the late 1910s and 1920s. The movement continued into the 1940s, especially as the war industries were desperate for labor. Introduction of the mechanical cotton picker after World War II, along with the increased use of tractors and other farm equipment, reduced the labor needs of southern agriculture even further.[64] Although none of this happened in an eyeblink, at some point, and again and again, the density of human population that was within flight range of thick clouds of anopheles fell below the critical level for continuing malaria transmission. The parasite's ecology was fragile to begin with; as the sharecropping cotton farmer disappeared from the rural South, malaria left as well.

Malariologist M. A. Barber described the requirements for the propagation of malaria in a population: "[T]he maintenance of high endemic malaria requires a permanent reservoir of infection such as is furnished by a considerable body of people lacking proper housing, proper food, and adequate medical treatment"[65] Once the sharecroppers moved away from the densest clouds of anopheles, the critical links in the continual malaria chain began to break down, one community at a time. Certainly other factors such as returning prosperity, drainage, pyrethrum sprays, and screening played their roles. But it was this removal of the malaria carrier/victim from the vicinity of the anopheles mosquito that probably had the largest effect on the decline in the plasmodium's presence.[66]

In this chapter we looked at the professionals and politicians of the 1930s, without giving much attention to the personal experience of malaria. The next chapter will attempt to remedy this deficit, mining a remarkable cache of interview material produced by the Works Progress Administration. The program may not have been very effective at malaria control, but its collection of southern oral histories allows insight into the health experiences of a broad swath of the southern population.

# Chapter 6

## Popular Perceptions of Health, Disease, and Malaria

Perhaps the hardest task faced by the medical historian is to understand how the patient, and not just the physician, experiences health and disease. The physician's perspective is easily accessible, in printed articles in medical journals and newspapers, testimony before legislative bodies, and reports of physician-staffed governmental agencies, as well as in diaries, letter books, and other personal documents. Physicians were both personally and professionally literate, and their *mentalité* is tidily cached for the digging historian. The narrative of this book so far has been derived from a profusion of such sources.

The patient is much harder to recover. The label *patient* is used in a self-consciously loose manner here, referring not only to a person who sees a health care practitioner for a particular complaint, but also to a community member who may be the target of public health education and practice. This broadening of the term is necessary to encompass the reality of health experience in the rural South, where many of the people who most interest the historian never actually became patients in the formal sense. Driven by the determination that the voiceless shall find a voice, explorers into medicine's past have eagerly sought remnants of the patient side of the physician-patient encounter. Most prior attempts to uncover the patient's point of view have focused on literate, affluent folks. Sheila Rothman's fine study of the impact of tuberculosis on a variety of nineteenth-century lives is exemplary; she is able to enter into the lives of her subjects precisely because they left letters or diaries behind.[1] Similarly Christopher Feudtner's work on the creation of diabetes as a chronic disease in the wake of insulin's therapeutic use draws heavily on the patient experience of this phenomenon. Again, though, the medium is the written document—in Feudtner's case, letters written to a physician who pioneered in diabetes care.[2] These two defining features, literacy and the ability to afford a doctor's attentions, have been hallmarks of at least modest affluence throughout most of American history.

There are a few ways through this curtain that separates us from the unspoken voices of the past, but none are entirely satisfactory. One way is to use a mirror, however distorted, to reflect a subject's point of view. Suppose a southern planter complains that his slaves are careless with tools, given to thieving, and prone to run away; his words may be mirroring something about the African slaves' patterns of resistance to white domination. The writings of physicians complaining about their patients' beliefs may provide similar mirrors of southern rural health perceptions for the early twentieth century. A second way through the curtain is demographic evidence. Where the data exist—in mortality rolls, parish records, ships' manifests—we can reconstruct something of the life of the individual. When we know that only half of those born into a community made it to adulthood, we can at least imagine that the reality of childhood mortality was a major emotional factor in its households. But we have to look elsewhere for evidence of how individual women and men coped with these recurring losses.

The most valuable tool for exploring the understanding of illiterate, historically remote people is the oral history interview. For recent history this tool is invaluable, as living minds recall past events, albeit with the usual caveats about the quirks and biases of memory. Unfortunately few such interviews exist for prior eras, and fewer still were done with any subjects but the elite. But the historian of medicine shares with southern historians in general a particularly rich cache of interviews done in the 1930s. Sponsored by the Federal Writers' Project (FWP) of the Works Progress Administration (WPA), these interviewers were explicitly instructed to seek out people from whom information about race and folk history could be elicited. The result was hundreds of interviews with some of the poorest of the South's poor, conducted during the later years of the Great Depression. Interviewers were told to inquire about health issues—providing, happily, grist for the medical historian's mill. The resulting narratives were composed not in the direct interview format but as stories, where the interviewer's presence is explicit but muted. Interviewers strove to let their subjects present themselves in their own words, although occasional background descriptions of the subject's appearance and habitat remind the reader of the presence of the observer.[3]

These sources should not be approached naïvely: the interviewers had no tape recorders, and the narratives are their reconstructions of conversations based on notes and recollection. Nor were they freestyle visits, for the interviewers had been instructed to ask a calendar of questions. Even the ways of transcribing dialect were prescribed, so that some consistency in recording would result. Only a few interviewers were black, and they achieved greater frankness in their interactions with rural African-Americans. Black southerners had long experience with telling white people what white people wanted to hear, which certainly colored the interviews. Further, many subjects clearly hoped that the WPA interviewer would be able to help them get relief, assuming that any white government person must have at least some influence with other white government persons. In spite of all these barriers to communication, these interviews are still the best inroad available into the rural southern mind of the 1930s.

The FWP interviewers toured the southern back roads at a time of great transition in southern history. They particularly sought out blacks who had memories of slavery, for that generation was rapidly passing. The late 1930s were a time when many African-Americans left the tenant culture of the rural South for town life, often traveling to northern cities for employment. Black girls took home economics classes in school, where they learned about diet and hygiene, only to go home to the care of grandmothers who still held to magic healing rituals. The radio, and soon the television, were entering this rural habitat, bringing with them a homogenization of thought that would soon eradicate most traces of the older folk culture that FWP interviewers were still able to record in 1937. They give us a glimpse of a culture that was fragmenting, reforming, assimilating the new, even while the old doggedly persisted. The historian can make few assured claims about what "the people," the "poor people," the "rural people," or the "rural black people" believed. No pollsters were active in 1937 to count how many of the inhabitants of Sunflower County, Mississippi, believed that malaria was caused by bad night air. But some clearly did, because such opinions were expressed in individual interviews, and because public health physicians persistently bewailed "the public's" ignorance.

My goal in this chapter is to try to show how the impoverished rural southerners who were most likely to get malaria understood not only this disease but illness, disease causation, and medical intervention in general. Thanks to the FWP interviews, we can catch glimpses into this complex array of perceptions. These interviews were undertaken as part of a self-conscious effort to get at "folk culture," the sort of sociological investigation perhaps best exemplified by Charles Johnson's work out of Fisk University in Nashville. Johnson's *Shadow of the Plantation* (1934) used interviews with rural black folk to describe the way of life in Macon County, Alabama, and included a valuable section on medical ideas.[4] His subjects were far from a pure "folk culture": they were no isolated New Guinea tribe discovered last month, with a coherent body of folk knowledge about the origin and structure of the universe and its parts. They had no single way to understand disease, for example; their explanations could include aspects of Christianity, nineteenth-century medical thought, magical thinking, and twentieth-century knowledge.

It is the very flexibility of this congregation that is so impressive, and that makes it so difficult to describe. A startling example comes from an interview with a black midwife from rural Alabama:

I gits a lot of herbs out there in the country where I lives and uses 'em fer a 'oman when she settin' in. They ain't got no money ter buy medicine. I biles 'em down and makes teas. . . . I never does sweep under a bed fer a 'oman laying in. Hit's bad luck. And when yer takes up de ashes, sprinkle 'em in front of de door. The best thing fer a 'oman laying in is a rabbit foot, fer luck. . . . I goes to the Medical Board every month and gives in how many chillun I kotch every month. . . . The best thing New-fallah is ever done is that Syphilis Clinic fer niggers. . . . I is a mid-wife and I knows all the idiot chillun, blind chillun, eczema chillun, deaf chillun an' a lot of other kine of ailments too comes 'cause their ma's has it. They didn't use ter know how to cure it, but they does now, ef you ain't too fur gone. Hit's awful how many niggers has it, but I don't believe it's as catching as folks says hit is; 'cause ef it wuz, everybody would have it. I sho' ain't careless though when I is around it. Ef I is with a 'oman that has it, I washes my hands with carbolic acid. Then I has them mercury tablets, little green ones, and I puts 'em in water and uses hit too.[5]

In this one remarkable passage, several systems of medical thought are represented. The woman knows about herbs that can be made into teas to ease childbirth. She believes in the magic of rabbits' feet and ashes properly laid down. She has empirical knowledge about the connection of syphilis and deformed children (she has seen it herself), and of the lack of easy contagion in syphilis. In her praise of the clinic's curative drugs, and the protective value of mercury and carbolic acid, she acknowledges the power of microbiology and modern pharmacology, although it is unclear whether she understood the action of these agents in the same terms as the doctors at the clinic. This midwife discovers no dissonance in holding these various perceptions simultaneously; that eclecticism is characteristic of the southern rural population featured in the WPA interviews.

Within any community of people, there were of course wide variations, as well as gradations of poverty and race. However poor, those living in "town" were more exposed to modern ideas and expectations, even when that "town" might consist of only five hundred or a thousand people. Although differences between blacks and whites were wide, differences within a single racial group mattered as well. Affluent urban whites were likely to hold different attitudes toward medicine and disease than the struggling sharecroppers of the same race. There was social stratification in the black community too, evident in comments about income, skin tone, behavior, education level, and rural/urban location. Thus any assignment of a single attitude or assumption to southern poor folks as a class runs a great risk of simplification. Still, none of these subgroups lived in isolation from each other, and their frequently expressed points of view probably had significance for at least a substantial minority of the population we are trying to explore.

While not minimizing these difficulties, this chapter will draw some broad conclusions about the southern rural individual's experience of disease and health in the first few decades of the twentieth century. In order to understand how malaria fit into this broader experience, the general patterns of disease causation and cure will be considered first, followed by an analysis of malaria's special place in popular conceptions of epidemiology. By the end of this chapter, the reader should have a new appreciation of the broad gulf between the mindsets of the scientifically trained public health physicians and the South's peasantry.

## The Naming and Origins of Illness

In any consideration of material drawn from interviews, the issue of translation looms large and immediate. Do the words used by the two people in question mean the same thing? Are they speaking the same language? FWP writers usually transcribed the speech of black subjects in dialect, indicating the interviewer's perception of differences between the standard English that the interviewer presumably spoke and the English of the subject. The interviewers were less prone to transcribe white speech in dialect—a disparity unlikely to have resulted from the total parity of their speech with that of college-educated Americans. Certainly FWP interviewers were interested in preserving "quaint" ways of expression among blacks and directly sought them out. This probably created a bias toward recording unusual labels rather than labels that were the same as the interviewer would have used. For example, when questioning one elderly black woman about her joint pains, the interviewer learned that the woman had seen a doctor. What had he given her for the arthritis? "Anna Jesus ba'm," she said proudly, and allowed that it had done some good. In case the reader missed the point, the interviewer put the words "analgesic balm" in parentheses following the statement.[6]

Aside from such whimsies, however, a great gulf remained between how the rural people of the South named and sorted their derangements of health and how the educated physician or layperson did so. Even the most sympathetic of interviewers, such as Charles Johnson, found that many people could characterize what was wrong with them only as "feeling kinda poorly" or "I ain't no good."[7] Johnson spoke of one family that suffered from an illness that they seemed to think was indigestion. Upon further inquiry, he acquired more details. "My boy's out there is sick. He got indijestus," said one saddened mother who had lost several children to this malady. "He'll start coughing and it hurts him all in there, and you kin hear him trying to git his breath and he just has that indijestus with it every time." Johnson concluded that the family's trouble was tuberculosis, but that inadequate diagnosis of the problem prevented any effective intervention. Another mother who had lost many children similarly dismayed him. "One eleven months old died with fever; one the thrase ran over him and one girl sixteen died in 1915. She got wet the wrong time. Doctor claim she had pellagacy."[8] Again the lack of communication between professional and patient is evident in this problem of naming. The mother knew the cause of illness to be an imbalance of moisture; the doctor was concerned about vitamin intake and pellagra. It was a classic case of "talking past each other" in which the participants appear to speak the same language but in effect are in such different worlds of understanding that communication is not possible.

Physicians no doubt at times thought they were being perfectly clear, and they were even adopting their patients' language. One now famous example occurred during the interviews for the Tuskegee syphilis study in the early 1930s. The physicians and other health professionals of the study defined syphilis as a disease caused by a spirochete, spread by sexual intercourse and childbirth, and curable by arsenic and mercury compounds. Their subjects, on the other hand, used a generic term of "bad blood" for certain sorts of illness. Although it is difficult to tell for certain in retrospect, the label "bad blood" likely included all the anemia diseases (including malaria and hookworm), and symptoms of malnutrition, as well as many cases of syphilis. And some blacks probably never used it at all. One Tuskegee subject recalled: "So I went on over and they told me I had bad blood." When asked by a historian if he knew that that meant syphilis, the man said, "That could be true. But I never heard no such thing. All I knew was that they just kept saying I had the bad blood—they never mentioned syphilis." The man was pleased that he was getting treatment for this condition, because they "gave me a blood tonic."[9]

Other disease categories could be just as puzzling to educated observers in the 1930s. One FWP interviewer met a woman on the street who was proudly carrying a bottle of "doctor's medicine." When asked what the trouble was, the woman reported, "Had the dissipate, Missus," a condition that had plagued her for on to five months.[10] Another woman mourned a child who had lived only eleven months and was now "dead with rheumonia."[11] Childhood complaints were frequently mysterious but were accepted with a certain fatalism. One woman had three children dead, of eleven born, one from a fight and one from whooping cough. Of the third death, she said, "Penny, she died in 1927. Po' chile, she jes' staid sick, complainin' wid her side an' stomach all de time. She stayed sick right round three years, den she died."[12] A farmer who talked to Charles Johnson described another complaint that is difficult to fit into any sort of modern disease category: "I was in the field plowing one day and I felt something jerkin' my head around. Then I tried to spit and I couldn't. . . . I been sick and not able to work for three years. I has miseries in my stomach."[13] It is easy to attribute such descriptions to ignorance, but in reality they represent an alternative way of organizing symptoms and events into an explanatory model of illness.

Part of the meaning attached to any disease label is the prognosis its name implies. Cancer carries a patina of horror because of its association with decay and death; rheumatism does not.[14] How a culture classifies illness as serious or trivial may change over time and may differ among social groups within a society. A modern example of this is high blood pressure, which may cause no symptoms for the patient but forebode heart disease and stroke when viewed through the medical professional's eye. Physicians working in the first third of the century struggled with like perplexities, especially those who worked among the rural southern folk. Even death might not be a convincing warning of the seriousness of a disease, as evidenced by one woman's comments regarding the loss of her husband. "He was allers saying he felt porely," she remembered. "What killed him I dunno; high blood pressure, the doctor said. 'Twant nothing serious what killed him."[15]

The cultural gap between doctor and patient became even more evident when the rural people talked about the causation of disease. Often their assumptions would have been concurrent with the medical opinion of the mid-nineteenth-century, prebacteriological era or even earlier. At other times their assumptions about etiology are clearly magical, seeing a disease as the outcome of wicked conjure, or a reduction in pain as the outcome of "sympathetic magic." Some illness was considered due to sin, and healing due to faith in God. Many explanations of disease thus blended together, along with a soupçon of modern medical thought. The drive to explain the origins of disease was strong, but the idea that mosquitoes or germs could be the relevant agents did not fit well into prevailing models of disease etiology.

Echoes of disease theory from prior centuries often appear in the FWP interviews. A common one was the idea that an emotionally startling experience for a pregnant woman could imprint her unborn child, an idea espoused by regular medicine well into the nineteenth century. One story told of a woman scared by a frog during pregnancy who bore a child with webbed feet.[16] Another common notion was that excess in food, drink, or exposure to the elements could cause illness. One woman attributed her abdominal symptoms to a fatty diet, for example. "Hit's my stomach," she explained. "You see I was the oldest of nine kids. We was powerful pore and it was mighty hard to feed so many. I et a lot of grease with my food and my stomach fought back. Hit finally loss the fight."[17] An elderly black woman in North Carolina, interviewed by an open fire on a warm day in June, expressed ideas of causation that reflected nineteenth-century medical thought exactly. When asked why she maintained the house so warm on a sunny day, the woman explained, "I got a misery in my chest. . . . And I'm scared to let in air a-comin' over new-plowed ground. It's agin good breathin'."[18]

"Misery" as a term for any discomfort or illness remains in common use among certain members of my own patient population, usually people who are black, or rural, or both. It expresses the most basic bodily awareness—something is wrong there, in that part. It hurts, or it does not work well, or both. Historians of medicine make much of the early modern movement from general theories of humoral imbalance to a localization of disease in organs or tissues, but the rural southern folk of the 1930s were not engaged by such subtleties. They had some understanding of what organs lay inside, if nothing else from the experience of butchering animals, and they could well believe that a heart or a lung or a stomach was not functioning as it should. But asking them to accept that microorganisms or mosquitoes were involved in disease causation was quite a stretch. It was easier to believe in the direct malevolence of conjure, or in the magical power of certain objects, as we shall see. Their incomprehension of the medical worldview was often evident in their attitudes toward regular medical therapeutics and public health efforts.

## Ways of Healing

Rural southerners had a variety of therapeutic options to choose from. Many men and women possessed knowledge of herbs that were known to have healing properties, or they might buy patent medicines to cure their symptoms. If accessible monetarily and spatially, a regular medical doctor could be called into attendance. Many communities had other healers as well. Some were self-professed conjure doctors, who mixed magic with herbal medicine. Others claimed that they were gifted to heal because God had called them, or they had been born with a caul that marked them as special. Midwives were abundant and at times expanded their practice to include herbal doctoring of nonparturient problems. Other practitioners were available with varying degrees of formal training—visiting public health nurses, chiropractors, and pharmacists—and might be called upon for advice and treatment. Then as now, allegiance to one sort of practitioner did not preclude seeking care from another. These were empirical-minded folk, who looked for medical care that was affordable and effective. Consistency with modern scientific thought was not one of their dominant criteria for judging treatment.

The most common form of medical care was self-treatment, which can be roughly divided into home remedies and patent medicines. Home remedies included herbs, which are frequently mentioned in the FWP narratives, and the application of such domestic substances as tar, kerosene, whiskey, and honey. From ex-slave narratives, it is clear that the herbal knowledge base had been continued through an oral tradition that extended to at least the antebellum era.[19] One ex-slave explained: "Where they was so many hands, bound ter be some of 'em sick right along. For dysentery, you make tea out of sweetgum buds; you get 'em way down in de leaves-like, an' make tea an' put a leetle flour in hit fer babies. Fer pneumonia, you make hog-hoof tea; take 'em off an' parch 'em an' pound hit up an' put hit in a bottle an' make tea. But you use sage tea fer fever. But, lor'! dat's what we does now when folks gits sick, twasn't jes in slavery time. Maybe hit started then—I don' know'm 'bout dat—but folks gits sick now same as they did then, an' we heals 'em de same way."[20] Many of the people represented in FWP interviews believed in the power of herbal and home remedies and were quick to say, "Doctors don't do so much good. Sometimes I think home-remedies are the best."[21]

The use of herbal remedies was often linked to religious belief and intermixed with prayer as a healing power. One woman admitted, "The Lord made medical doctors, but I don't believe in 'em." She went on to proclaim her faith: "What's herbs for? I've doctored with 'em sixty years. The Lord put herbs here, and everything's got a purpose. . . . As for herbs, what better medicine do you want? The Lord put 'em here to doctor the pore that couldn't buy store medicine."[22] One Virginia black man was likewise proud of his healing power, which he attributed in fairly equal parts to his earthly and heavenly fathers. "My daddy knew all de roots an' he showed dem to me," he explained. "I just go an' get me some roots when ever I feel sick. I know master weed, peter's root, may apple, sweet william roots are good for a lot of things. . . . Dere's a root for ev'y disease an' I can cure most anything, but you have got to talk wid God an' ask him to help out."[23] Both of these speakers were quite old in the 1930s, and the extent to which their knowledge was accepted by younger members of their family is difficult to know. But enough consciousness of herbal remedies remained that two researchers culling the Georgia WPA interviews for herbal medications found more than ninety different herbs described, along with their medicinal purposes.[24]

Herbal potions were widely used by conjurors as well, and it is worth digressing a bit to explore the place of magic in the WPA narratives. The interviewers were specifically instructed to seek information on the subject, and in some places they led the witnesses egregiously. "Does hearing a hoot owl mean some one is going to die?" they asked each subject, and all the person being interviewed had to say was yes or no. Much of the discussion of signs and amulets reflected not the prominence of this knowledge in the speaker's mind but the eagerness of the interviewer to elicit such information. If we factor in the desire of those interviewed to please the FWP writers, then we conclude that at least some of the abundant material on superstition must be discounted. Still, there are accounts so detailed, so convincing that they have to be taken seriously.[25]

Although individual laypersons might know a few techniques of magic, such as wearing lucky amulets and making certain signs to ward off evil, most magical healing was done by professionals. Some limited their activity to curing disease and might be more accurately termed "root doctors." A rural Virginia woman recorded one such person: "De conjure doctor, old Dr. Jones, walk 'bout in de black coat like a preacher, and wear sideburns, and use roots and sich for he medicine. He larnt 'bout dem in de piney woods from he old granny. He didn't cast spells like de voodoo doctor, but used roots for smallpox, and rind of bacon for mumps, and sheepwool tea for whoopin' cough. . . . He could break conjure spells with broth."[26] Although this man's practice was benign, other conjure practitioners would create evil, for a price, sometimes with the same herbs used for healing. One Georgia man defined the practice of conjuring this way, after admitting to believing in its powers: "Yes, man, I knows 'bout conjurs—plenty o' conjurs. Dem conjur-folks takes weeds and yerbs, and fixes you so you can't sleep and can't eat and bark like a dog."[27]

The practice of conjuring appears to have used, besides herbs, less obviously medicinal compounds to cast spells as well. An elderly Virginia woman revealed what she had learned about conjure practices: "[O]ne told me that it was easy for folks to put snakes, frogs, turtles, spiders, or most anythin' . . . on the inside of you. He said these things was killed and put up to dry and then beat up into dust. If any of this dust is put in somethin' you have to eat or drink, these things will come alive like they was eggs hatchin' in you."[28] Such practices built on common knowledge for their plausibility—tiny seeds grow into big plants, little eggs into big creatures—and were more believable than some of contemporary public health doctrine. Other magical practices included using the clothing or other personal items of the person bewitched. Many charms were "worked" in order to secure a person's affections, get a job, or otherwise affect someone's judgment.

To all appearances, conjurer and conjured alike believed in the power of such magic. One woman told the sad story of her son's ill health, with all sincerity: "I got a son . . . well somebody fixed him. . . . He would squeal jest like a pig and he would get down on his knees and bark jest lak a dog." She took her son to a conjure doctor, who confirmed that the boy was bewitched and offered to treat him. "Then he took Jack in a room took off his clothes and started ter rubbing him down with medicine all the same time, he wuz saying a ceremony over him, then he took them 8 dimes put 'em in a bag and tied them around Jacks Chest some where so that they would hang over his heart." After noting that this treatment resulted in Jack's recovery from near death, his mother laments that "Jack wore them dimes a long time but he finally drunk 'em up."[29] The modern skeptic might wonder if alcohol caused Jack's symptoms in the first place, but the elderly woman telling this story doubtless had faith in the conjure doctor's explanation and cure of her son's disease.

Even white women would go to black doctors who were felt to have special knowledge and power over disease. Much like alternative healers today, such practitioners had a patina of power in the absence of harsh measures such as surgery. One white female coal miner in Alabama told of her encounter with such a doctor:

> I've heard so much talk about sickness and operations that I even got to thinking that the pain in my legs and back wasn't rheumatism, maybe, so I decided to go to a doctor, myself, but not one of those doctors that work at a hospital, where it's so handy just to step in and operate. I heard about a fine Negro doctor up in the country that just tells what's the matter with you. . . . I went in and he . . . looked at my fingernails and then at my eyeballs. Then he told me I didn't have rheumatism like I thought I did, but I had female trouble—whatever that is, I don't know. This doctor gave me four quarts of terrible smellin' herb medicine and it tasted as bad as it smelled. He told me to come back when all my medicine was gone and that'll be next Saturday. I feel fine already and I sleep lots better.[30]

Whatever he did appeared to the patient to work, which is all that it takes to convince a person of a practitioner's power.

A few of the conjure doctors themselves were interviewed by the FWP writers. While their accounts may well be biased in the direction of hiding cultural information from the white person or exaggerating the extent of exotic behavior to titillate the hearer, they are the best we have and remain a valuable resource about how such healers acted. One Alabama man summarized his conjure career as follows: "I quit loadin' cross-ties, an' move to Montgomery, whar I open a lil Shop as Herbdoctor, Fortune-teller, an' Conjure-man. I soon stop foolin' wid herbs dou'. Dey wahn't nuff money in dat fur me. Niggers won't pay but half dollar fur no herb medicine. But dey'll spen' five or ten dollars fur to git somebody conjured. Dey'll go on payin' too, munt after munt, yer after yer fur to keep dat spell fasten on some po' pusson what dey hates. . . . I has a nice lil income out of de palsy, rheumatic pains, chills an' fever, coughin' fits, an' sudden misery what I sends on folks to pacify dey enemies. Besides all dat, I charge fifty cents a week to keep de sickness on 'em after hit's once ketch holt."[31] The man was proud of his skills, and when questioned about his ethical propriety, he said that he had his job to do in society just like lawyers and police. He was assured a place in heaven and even sketched for the interviewer his fantasy of arriving in glory.

Other magical workers shunned practices that caused harm and focused their efforts mostly on healing. Specialization by disease was not unusual. One elderly man's only medical skill was that he could make bleeding stop. A North Carolina healer could cure thrash, an infantile throat malady, because she had never seen her father.[32] Others had knowledge of particular remedies for particular ailments. Venereal diseases were a common target of such secret potions. When one rural southerner failed to be cured of gonorrhea by shots from a regular doctor, he went to another authority. "Now I'm taking a medicine from a nigger at Paris, [Tennessee,] Lucian Freeman—he's a barber. I pay him five dollars a bottle for it," he told the interviewer. "The bottles ain't labeled so I don't know what's in it. . . . It's brown stuff and smells like turpentine and has some old stringly white stuff in it like the white of an egg. Yes, it sure does taste awful, but I sort of believe it's a-doing me some good, though."[33]

It was a short step from privately produced remedies to patent medicines, which were enormously popular throughout the United States in the 1930s. In that decade around 10 percent of each health care dollar was spent on patent medicine purchases, and this proportion was higher in the South.[34] Perhaps the most pervasive was the "black draught" used for constipation.[35] Rural southerners bought patent medicines from traveling salesmen, from local stores, and by sending away for items advertised on the radio.[36] Local people also sold patent medicines to their friends as a way to raise extra money, much as "Avon ladies" would in later years. One FWP interviewer witnessed such an encounter. While the interviewer was in the home of Sally, an interview subject, a neighbor dropped by to announce that the company was giving away dish towels this week, one for every dollar of merchandise ordered. Sally declined the offer.

> "'Twon't be nothin' for me this week, Mrs. Flack. Ruth has took all that cough medicine she got from you but that little bit up there in the bottle, but it ain't seemed to do her no good at all." Mrs. Flack raised her eyes to the mantel to look at the almost empty bottle. "It is nearly gone," she said. "Better let me leave you another bottle."
> "No, I reckin not this time," Sally responded.[37]

Failing in this sale, Mrs. Flack also tried to sell Sally some vanishing cream, but she wasn't having any. Aside from the evident inefficacy of Mrs. Flack's products, Sally was limited by her empty purse. Even though patent medicines were cheaper than care from a physician, they still made a dent in the budget.

## Calling a Physician

There were, of course, conventional physicians in the rural South, and patients who sought their care. The popularity of various alternative modes
of healing should not obscure the fact that scientific medicine was not only
represented in the South but had an unavoidable impact on how the rural
people thought about health and disease. Scientific medicine was not the
only system to which they turned, but it was a major influence. Still, there
were barriers between the physician and the rural patient. The most immediate barrier was cost, but geography and distrust also separated doctors
and patients. Yet, as Charles Johnson tells us, almost half of the 612 black
families in Macon County, Alabama, used the services of a physician in
1931.[38] This figure shows that rural blacks expected regular medicine to
have significant value for them, and that some ways must have been worked
out for this impoverished population to afford medical care. A black man
summed up this dilemma in 1937, after exhaling a stream of tobacco smoke:
"I owe the doctor right smart already and can't pay him. I ain't got no
health. I have asthmie so bad some nights I don't sleep a wink. . . . I have
to go the doctor three and four times some weeks, and sometimes he has
to come here. . . . I keep capsules here all the time for emergency, but they
ain't as good as hypode'mics."[39] He thus simultaneously admitted an in-
ability to pay, the continued attendance of the doctor, and the superior
efficacy of modern medical care. These are all important factors in understanding how regular medicine was integrated into southern rural culture.

Many families, white and black, lived in such destitution that a doctor
was an unaffordable luxury, not a basic need on the order of having enough
to eat. One dismayed FWP interviewer vividly recorded the condition of a
two-room farmhouse that was home to nine people: "The floor, in which
big cracks admit damp air from under the house, is stained with grease
spots and snuff-dipping. Flies swarm around two green 'possum hides that
hang in the hall. A stench of unwashed bodies, tobacco juice burned on
dog-irons, rats' nests, squalor is over all. . . . 'We don't have the doctor
here,' [said the brood's mother,] 'They's nothin' to pay with; so what's the
use to send for him? All we can do when we get sick is to tough it out best
we can.'"[40] A black man went so far as to claim that slavery was better than
freedom, because at least a man got health care then. "Sometimes ah think
slavery wuz bettuh den freedom in one sense," he mused. "Ef ye wuz sick,
ye hadda doctuh. . . . But now ef ye git sick an' ye hain' got no money, ye
jis die. Dat's all!"[41]

Certainly doctors could and did refuse to take cases when no money
was forthcoming. This was particularly true in obstetrics cases, perhaps
on the assumption that the baby would get born some way or other, often
with the help of a midwife. When a North Carolina woman described the

log cabin existence of her childhood, she recalled: "Mam was sick all the time. . . . We was too pore to have doctors. When Linnie was borned I won't only seven but I helped the nigger woman fetch her."[42] A twenty-seven-year-old woman pregnant with her eleventh child described a difficult delivery that might have ended in death without a doctor's presence, although her husband had a terrible time getting a doctor to come. "Before Dr. Boster started treating me I nearly died," her saga began. "Rudolph called up four doctors and none of them would come to see me. They said Rudolph . . . could have made arrangements for one of them to take care of me, and that he could have paid them a little money along. Then they would have been glad to have taken care of me." Rudolph was out of work, and the only way they got a doctor was to have the mayor intercede in their behalf.[43]

When families did go into debt to pay for medical care, it could destroy what prosperity they had. After housing, food, and the materials necessary for farming, medical care was the major economic cost, and one that was so unpredictable. In families that tottered continually on the brink of destitution, medical bills could thoroughly ruin them. One woman turned to prostitution in order to pay her child's hospital bills and care for him.[44] Another man blamed his desperate poverty on medical expenses. "When my wife died I was in good shape financially," he remembered. "I didn't owe a cent, and I had five bales o' cotton on hand. It took them five bales to pay the doctors' bills and her burial expenses, and I begin then to get behind."[45]

Patients had to deal not only with doctors but sometimes with the hospital, the home nurse, costly medicines, and even the altered diet ordered by the doctor. Increasingly, rather than dispensing medicines directly, physicians were writing prescriptions that had to be taken to the pharmacy. And increasingly they were sending patients to the hospital for surgery, difficult deliveries, and serious medical conditions. With recent discoveries about vitamins, especially the role of niacin in preventing pellagra, physicians were often in the position of recommending a diet that patients could not afford. Eggs, milk, meat, and vegetables—all rich in niacin and other vitamins—were simply too expensive to put on the table regularly. One fatalistic woman described just such a situation regarding her daughter: "Mary has some sorter dizzy spells every two or three months and we have to send her to the hospital. The doctor prescribed a diet for her, but we ain't able to give her the food that she ought to have."[46] Given poverty as profound as this, the doctor's advice was ultimately of little value.

Geographical barriers compounded the problems. The miserable state of southern rural roads made travel by horseback the only practical transport at times. More and more doctors refused to make house calls in the country, for the time and effort involved was rarely covered by what the patient could pay. Indeed one North Carolina farmer planned to move his whole family so that medical care would be more accessible. "That's what I want to do, move on a farm about a mile from town so if we have to have the doctor it won't take half a month's wages to pay him. Here where we are, thirteen mile from Emporia and nine from Seaboard, a doctor won't come for less than six dollars, and he's got to know the money's here waitin' for him at that. It's so inconvenient to get a doctor too. When the creek's up, there's no gettin' to Seaboard for nothin', and the road's sandy and crooked at the best. There's no telephone in this country. I have to get somebody to go all the way to Emporia after a doctor—thirteen miles there and thirteen miles back."[47] The glib phrase "Lord willin and the creek don't rise," which modern southerners are apt to spout when confirming an invitation, had real meaning to rural people in the 1930s, when the ability to get to a doctor made the difference between life and death.

Aside from poverty and geography, race was an obvious barrier to health care. Hospitals were openly segregated until the 1960s, and the quality of medical services available at the black hospitals was notoriously inferior.[48] Race is less prominent in the WPA narratives (although the documents themselves always make clear whether the subject is black or white). Certainly physicians maintained segregation in their outpatient clinics past midcentury. I can well remember seeing the sign on the "colored waiting room" at my own doctor's office in Paris, Tennessee, during the 1960s. But the physicians and patients interviewed by the WPA do not talk about access to health care being limited by race, and indeed physicians were apt to boast that they good-heartedly took care of everybody. They may have categorized patients more by class and promptness of bill paying than by skin color, for this subject is far more prominent in the available documents. But race was always a factor, even if it was not discussed openly in polite company.

Given that doctors needed a livelihood and people needed health care, ways to facilitate this interaction without cash were found. Barter was common; my Tennessee grandfather accepted chickens and other farm produce in lieu of cash for dental services. One North Carolina physician, who recounted that he had been paid in everything from antique furniture to brandy, cited two particularly remarkable instances of "payment in kind." In one case he took two hundred plow beams, although he had little use for such an abundance. But he drew the line at another: "One mother whom I had attended at the birth of her six children, without being paid, called me in for her seventh delivery. After it was all over and she was comfortable, she looked up at me and said, with the utmost sincerity: 'Dr. Cain, I've never been able to pay you nothin' for deliverin' my other six children; so I'll give you this one.' I didn't tell her I'd rather deliver six more for her free, than to accept this 'fee.'"[49] Dr. Cain and other physicians also reported that they did much medical work for free, because they knew their patients and knew that, at least temporarily, the patients couldn't pay. "Pay? Pshaw!" an Alabama doctor sputtered. "These people can't pay. But they used to [pay]. . . . I haven't spent all of that [money] yet."[50]

One traditional way of having health care paid for was by private charity. This often took the form of employer-employee philanthropy. A man who worked in an Alabama sawmill, for example, needed a cataract operation to restore his sight and his fitness to work. His employer paid for it.[51] Elderly black women frequently found patrons among middle-class whites, especially ones they had worked for as domestics or to whom they had some other tie. Mandy Johnson, a black midwife born in 1867, explained to the FWP interviewer how she got along. "De way I lib now is jes' wid Rosie, dis here daughter workin' for Miss Labuzan, an', too, Miss Labuzan is allus sendin' me things. When I gits sick she gits me medicine."[52] A landlord might extend this sort of medical philanthropy to his or her tenants. In one case the landlord doctored the sick tenants directly, in the mode of the plantation master or mistress dosing the slaves. In another, though, the landlord boasted that "I provided medical attention for my tenants whenever they need it and generally the bill runs into several hundred dollars each year."[53]

It is difficult to know how often such care was provided, or whether it was provided gratis or taken out of the tenants' pay. Anger against landlords for their miserly ways frequently shone through the WPA interviews. In describing her condition, an elderly South Carolina sharecropper moaned, "I'se jes' 'bout nekkid myse'f, but I kin meck out summers. Hit's dese heah grandchillen what frets me." As her story continued, the complex web of the southern "safety net" became evident. "I went down to de relief place what gives clothes an' sich truck, an' de lady what run de she-bang ax me effen Mister Stores [the landlord] doan' teck kere of he han's, an' I tole her, 'No, mam, dat he sho' doan't!' She knowed right well I wuz tellin' de Gawd's truth, an' her eyes kinda flash lak, an' she sez: 'Damn em, dey wucks de po' niggers an' white buckra mos' to death in de spring an' summer, and fall, an' den loads em on us after stealin' dere share de crop! An' den dey got de nerve to cuss de relief! Why! *dey's* de ones meckin' money offen de guvment! Damn em!' "[54] Southerners disliked federal interference and any implication that they did not "take care of their own," but the plain truth was that the southern rural poor frequently did without essential food, shelter, and health care.

Southerners were not entirely bereft, however, when it came to paying doctors' bills. Some invested in insurance schemes to help with the costs. One woman who worked at Penney's department store reported that she and her co-workers had formed a medical insurance association.[55] Although Southerners far more commonly bought insurance to guarantee that the costs of burial were paid for, some companies would cover medical needs for a fee (and if the payments were kept up religiously). A twenty-five-year-old Macon, Georgia, woman bought medical insurance for herself and her husband from two insurance companies. "Both of us pay a dollar a month to both of them," she explained. "They pay us five dollars a week if we get sick and a hundred dollars at death. I was sick about a month ago, was sick and had to be away from my job for two weeks but I was behind on one of my policies. The one I was behind with jest paid me $2.50 but the other one paid me all right. It sure was a help but the doctor charged me three dollars every time he came and I didn't have enough for him and all the medicine I had to buy, too. Since I've been back at work I've 'bout gotten everything paid up though."[56] Her insurance did not pay much, but it helped her through the time of not only medical bills but also no paycheck.

Other folks worked out some sort of scheme of credit or payroll deduction. This was particularly true of those poor southerners who nonetheless collected a regular salary, the cotton mill workers. "Three year ago Iry had a operation fer rupture and it cost him $150. Hit looked like he'd never git that one paid fer," said one North Carolina woman. "Robert Hall [the boss at the cotton mill] had made the arrangements at the hospital and when Iry went back to work he took out so much a week. Tain't been long neither since he stopped takin' out fer it."[57] Another stooped old man who worked at a mill in Greensboro, North Carolina, was cursed with an invalid wife, a daughter who was hospitalized multiple times for "sinus" and a son with a "leakage of the heart." He just stayed in debt to the hospital. In an attempt to get the WPA interviewer to intercede for him with the welfare office, he detailed the sad state of his finances: "Three dollars goes for help every week, two dollars to the hospital,—I signed up to pay that much and the company just takes it out of my pay—ninety-four cent a week for house rent . . . [and] they ain't a week passes I don't spend from two to three dollars for the old lady's medicine."[58] He managed all this on $24.00 a week, the combined wages of himself and his son. Some textile mills actually maintained a company physician to keep their employees in good health, but even then the workers had to pay prescription costs.[59]

A final barrier that stood between rural southern patients and physicians was suspicion. Modern doctors used techniques that were unfamiliar and frightening. Even when the doctor was accessible and made a house call, the visit could be highly unsatisfactory for the patient. One South Carolina man reminisced fondly about old-style medicine and then explicitly disparaged modern physicians:

> [Old Dr. Moseley] comes and sets wid me fer an hour or mo',
> and he has his pill box wid him, and he measures me out some
> pills and feels de beating of my pulse in my wristes. Soon I

becomes better. I like Dr. Moseley, kaise he is old and he don't never be in no great rush. Young doctors comes and says, "howdy" and shakes something shiny in de light of de winder, and tells you to open your mouth; and dat shiny thing goes in and stays a while. Den dey takes it out and looks at it and writes on a piece of paper and den dey gives you de paper and says, "Goodbye." Of course you has to send somebody to Union to de drug sto' whar dat paper gits you some medicine. If you was much sick, you would lay down and die afo' a lazy young nigger could git back wid it fer you.[60]

He could no longer share a common understanding of illness and its treatment with these newer doctors, and he also worried that in his helplessness he might die due to dependency on others.

Young doctors, modern doctors, and student doctors were particularly to be feared, with their strange technology and tendency toward surgery. An elder Tennessee woman's tentative encounter with a physician showed both suspicion and autonomy in physician-patient interactions: "This leg got hurt. . . . [T]he white folks would say, 'Aunt Lizzie, . . . [w]hy don't you go to the doctor?' and I say, 'I don't want to go see any of those students, they will cut on me.' . . . So I went to a doctor in East Nashville, and I told him to bind it so it be all right. I told him he had bound it too tight yesterday. My leg was swollen up, and when I came home and got the scissors and cut it, and my leg got all right."[61] She retained control and certainly knew exactly what she wanted, regardless of the diagnosis or therapeutic advice of her doctors. Yet she did go to see one, a not-uncommon release of partial control in return for the possible improvement of a bad health situation.

Fears of medical experimentation did not begin with the 1972 revelations about the Tuskegee project. Poor southerners, and especially poor black southerners, had long experienced a loss of autonomy at the hands of doctors that created suspicion, especially about surgery. One woman whose child had bad tonsillitis acknowledged, "Doctors told me to have them took out," but she averred, "I'd heap rather see one of mine dead than in the hospital."[62] A Mississippi man attributed the area's poor health care in part to hospital phobia. "In dis day folks lays a bed ailen en poorly en all dey gits is some no count patent medicine." Why? "Dey is 'fraid to go to de horspital cause de doctahs might cut on dey stummicks."[63] Another elderly black man reported that he had even been at risk of being abducted by physicians, equating their tactics with the Ku Klux Klan. "De only Ku Klux I ever bumped into was a passel o' young Baltimore Doctors tryin' to ketch me one night an' take me to de medicine college to 'periment on me," he claimed.[64] Modern physicians had power but also the potential for harm, and they were to be approached only with the greatest caution.

The medical world of the rural southerner in the early twentieth century was a complex place. Disease could be caused by a neighbor's jealous conjuration, an ill wind, a germ, or too much grease. A single indisposition might be cured by an herbal potion, swallowing kerosene, visiting a magical healer, or going to the hospital. The patient rarely shared the understanding of disease causation and classification of the physician, much less the physician's allegiance to science as the arbiter of health knowledge. Rather, the focus was on the empirically experienced effectiveness of therapy, which was frequently modified by the family's ability to afford the treatment. It was into this mesh of health beliefs that physicians seeking to control malaria stepped, and which led to their frustrated outbursts against the ignorance and superstition of the people. In the next section we shall see this encounter, first from the perspective of physicians and public health workers, and then from that of the southern people who heard their peculiar message about the mosquito's relevance to chills and fever.

### The Public Health Professionals Encounter Malaria

"Our first effort in malaria control has been and, I am afraid, will for a long time continue to be, a striving to eradicate firmly cherished delusions concerning the disease itself and the methods of its transmission," the state health officer of Virginia moaned at a conference in 1922. "It would be rather amusing, if it were not so depressing, to note the many who refuse to consider the mosquito at all in connection with the disease, but attribute the whole trouble to night air. . . . That and the delusion about sewer gas are the most difficult to dispel," he despaired. He then listed all the causes of malaria that people had to be told not to believe—eating certain fruits, breaking the sabbath, or other ideas that he considered superstitious.[65] This public health official found the people to be ignorant and stubborn about their established beliefs.

A great gulf loomed between the educated physician engaged in public health work and the rural population. The tendency of the former to sneer at the latter did not make communication any easier. Oscar Dowling, of the Louisiana State Board of Health, told the following story, evidently identifying with the public health educator:

> Dr. Hurty, of Indiana, relates an experience apropos. He felt much encouraged at what he deemed an enthusiastic meeting of farmers to discuss ways and means for the elimination of typhoid fever. After going over the minutest details of prevention in the plainest language, one old farmer got up, and . . . "combed a pint of manure out of his beard with his fingers, and with great deliberation, said, 'Now, we don't believe a word of that stuff you've been telling us, and you don't believe it either,'

and evidently he voiced the sentiments of the crowd." Though ninety per cent refuse to be taught, it is worth while to teach the ten remaining. The young mind presents the most helpful soil in which to plant the seed which shall grow into a goodly tree of sanitary knowledge.[66]

Dowling drew on the tale to illustrate not just ignorance but skepticism. The populace did not trust either the knowledge given or the knowledge giver.

This suspicion often emerged in antimosquito work. During the 1905 yellow fever epidemic in New Orleans, when city workers went around oiling water barrels in the immigrant section, they were set upon by mobs who feared that the oil was poison.[67] State health workers in Tennessee reported that farmers would not believe that kerosene spread on ponds was harmless to stock. One farmer lost five cows and brought suit against the kerosene-spreaders.[68] Gaining public trust was even harder when the people had to be convinced not just that malaria was spread by mosquitoes but that mosquitoes bred in still water. "This statement of error was made by a public official in a small town before a group which was considering a drainage and general mosquito control program," said a North Carolina malaria worker. "'All this talk about mosquitoes coming from these swampy areas is the bunk. I know that mosquitoes come from China berry trees and the hedges around the yards, and I say to cut down the China berry trees and we won't have the mosquitoes.'" The same gentleman was sure that "'as for getting rid of malaria. I eat plenty of hog meat and peas and have never had malaria.'"[69] The local man's argument was accepted over that of the outsider, and no antimosquito work was done. Even those who accepted that the mosquito was involved did not always get all the details right. "A man was explaining to me just how the mosquito became infected," continued the North Carolina public health official. "'The mosquito when it hatches from the water sips up some of that green skim which you see on them ditches and then flies to someone and bites him. . . . [I]t injects some of this skim into the person and he gets malaria.'"[70]

This ignorance occurred against a larger background of sanitary innocence. Malaria fighters despaired of transmitting the complex mosquito story when even the simplest rules of hygiene were scoffed at. For example, an educated and self-consciously superior black man explained the attitude of his neighbors about personal cleanliness: "Some of de niggers here 'bouts don't wash but once a week. If you say anything to 'em about it dey'll tell you pretty quick dat dey is black and dirt don't show on 'em like it does on white folks."[71] This cavalier attitude was especially prevalent about toilets. Few rural southerners of either race had access to plumbing, so if they had a constructed toilet at all, it was a structure with a bench, situated at best over a hole in the ground. Was there a toilet on her place? one FWP interviewer asked a rural black woman. "None a-tall," she said, "jes a back house; not much account either. I usually go down in that big gully there, it saves hiring that back house moved."[72] Outhouses had to be maintained, and often tenants and landlords neglected that task. "Mister Stores, he is sho' one hard man to wuck for, yassuh, dat he sho' is," lamented a South Carolina sharecropper. "We ain' even got no toilet no mo. De ole un is fell down, an' Mister Stores he won't put up a new 'un. De guvment man come out an' sez he kin put up one what de relief mens is meckin' fo' ten dollars. But Mister Stores, he jes' laugh an' sez, 'Let em go to de bushes lak dey been er-doin'.'"[73] This anecdotal evidence is reinforced by the data gathered by hookworm campaigners, who demonstrated the general lack of even the most primitive hygiene facilities in the rural South.[74]

Public health officials saw the population not just as ignorant but as apathetic. Malaria was one of several "invisible diseases" that had to be brought into the light of day. Hookworm had been the first of these diseases to be illuminated and seen. Indeed, the first challenge of public health reformers fighting hookworm had been to convince the southern middle classes, including physicians, that the disease was there at all. The fatigue and weakness that followed hookworm were seen more as a way of life (and often as a mark of the lazy lower classes) than as symptoms of a specific disease. Reformers also struggled to highlight pellagra, to make it a fixable public health problem and not just a common condition of the underprivileged. With malaria, a similar pattern emerged. First, physicians had to be trained to recognize and treat malaria properly, as well as to take it seriously. The people, too, had not only to be taught about the disease's cause and cure but also to be aroused as to its importance. C. C. Bass, the physician who thought so highly of quinine as a community cure for malaria, encapsulated this barrier to reform: "Malaria is such an insidious disease that it is generally considered lightly, as a necessary evil of little importance, by those who live in localities where it prevails."[75] A USPHS physician demonstrated equal frustration in his attempts to raise the populace's consciousness about malaria when he remarked, "The negroes accept 'chills' as a necessary evil and pay it scant attention."[76] One of his colleagues echoed this sentiment, expanding it to both races: "The one obstacle to malaria control in the United States is our ignorant and therefore indifferent classes, both white and black. . . . [O]ur poorer people remain in the mire of ignorance."[77]

Education, especially of impressionable children, was the answer for such general ignorance and apathy, proclaimed the public health gospel underlying both the hookworm and the malaria efforts. For example, in 1920 North Carolina schoolchildren had the opportunity to compete for $25.00 prizes by writing winning essays on malaria and its control.[78] Public health officials widely believed that children could be convinced of their message even if adults remained skeptical and uncooperative. A Georgia malaria campaigner reported in 1925, "Two years ago in my rounds the children told me things like these: 'We get malaria from dirty ponds, night air, sugar cane, fish in stale water, watermelons in dog days, flies and mosquitoes raised in weeds, pea vines, trees.'" Now, he was proud to announce, they knew all about larvae, stagnant water, and the effect of oil on breeding grounds. "We are rapidly growing a population that will demand health appropriations large enough to do some practical prevention."[79] This appeal to the younger generation was easily made through the school system, and even if their parents continued to scoff, the inevitable passage of years brought more and more aware southerners to adulthood.

## *The Rural Perception of Malaria*

Many rural southerners did not think in terms of malaria as such: they had "chills" and used remedies for "chills," uninterested in differentiating their maladies further. Thus Zora Neale Hurston's folk-tale account of the origin and prevention of chills made sense, without any resource to medical thinking. Hurston had gathered such stories among Depression-era African-Americans in Florida and recorded them in her own inimitable style. She heard the following account from one man:

> "When you git yo' chear all set where you wants it, then you walk up to de mantel piece and turn yo' back to de fire—dat's to knock de breezes offen yo' back. You know, all de time youse outside in de weather, li'l breezes and winds is jumpin' on yo' back and crawlin' down yo' neck, to hide. They'll stay right there if you don't do somthin' to git shet of 'em. They don't lak fires, so when you turn yo' back to de fire, de inflamed atmosphere go up under yo' coat-tails and runs dem winds and breezes out from up dere. Sometimes, lessen you drive 'em off, they goes to bed wid you. Ain't y'all never been so you couldn't git warm don't keer how much kivver you put on?"
>
> "Many's de time I been lak dat."
>
> "Well," went on Dad, "Dat because some stray breezes had done rode you to bed."[80]

Both Hurston and the people she studied classed this sort of story among tall tales and clearly vied with each other to tell yet a more outrageous whopper. So it would be naïve to take these stories at face value and view them as part of a serious set of origin myths. On the other hand, it is illustrative that "chills" assumes a reified state here, at least enough to deserve its own origin myth, however far-fetched.

Once a problem had been diagnosed as "chills," it was logical to take a chill tonic. This conclusion seemed straightforward, and sales of chill tonics supported its widespread popularity. For example, one black woman from North Carolina reported scornfully after a physician had evaluated her child, "The doctor says he's got bromical pneumonia." But she knew better. "I looked at the child a few minutes and then says: 'The doctor's a bromical lie! That child's had a chill 'swhat ails him.' I went to work on him with chill tonic, and by the next day he was settin' up in a chair, wropped up in a bedquilt."[81] Consequently, anything that could be treated with such a tonic was not serious enough for a doctor's attention. A South Carolina WPA interviewer said of the black section of one South Carolina town, "Medical attention is practically unheard of in the Barondel Street." There were midwives for deliveries, of course: "Except for 'de fever' with which every Negro resident is stricken now and again, there is no illness, and who ever heard of going to a doctor for 'de fever'?" Instead, "everybody knows that you just have to find 25 cents for a bottle of 'RRR'!"[82]

E. W. Grove made a fortune off his chill tonic by promising that it was so sweet-tasting that babies would smile after taking it, but most southerners associated the effectiveness of quinine with its bitter taste. Some called quinine "old-fashioned," which, given its early-nineteenth-century pedigree, it certainly was.[83] Others compared bitter herbs to quinine and claimed their effectiveness. One South Carolina man reported, "Me and Mr. Sexton made tea from 'grance grey beard leaves to bust up chills. It act and taste jest like Quinine."[84] An Alabama woman offered her grandmother's remedy for chills, its effectiveness again attested to by its bitterness: "Take nine bitter weed flowers and boil them in three tablespoons of water. You give one teaspoon full of this at a time and it will break fever and chills, when nothin' else won't. It ought to, fer no quinine could be as bitter."[85]

Even the name *malaria* seems to have incompletely penetrated southern rural consciousness. As a label it was fairly new, almost as new as the concept that mosquitoes cause the disease. An exchange on a front porch in Marion, North Carolina, was telling:

> "Don't go until Ruth brings the baby," Ethel said. "She'll be
> here before long, I know."
> "I hope she ain't took it down to Terry's pa's. They might let
> a mosquito bite it and hit'd have malarial like Terry's mama has
> had this summer."
> "It's malaria, mama," Blanche said.
> For just a second Mamie looked embarrassed. Then she said,
> "Well, malaria, I reckin that is right."[86]

It is not accidental that the teacher in this case was the child, and the learner the adult. The public health message was penetrating via the younger generation. Older names persisted as well, along with the frequent mentions of chills and fever. "Us is all strong folks," said Lou, a turpentine worker in Stapleton, Alabama. "We ain't never needed no medicine 'ceptin when de boy had 'lignant fever. Boss Man sent down some quinine and Boy is good now."[87]

Skepticism about the mosquito's role in disease transmission was widespread, with age and gender influencing acceptance. Women paid more attention to health matters and were more prone to learn lessons from their children who attended health lectures at school. "The mosquitoes worry us pretty much in the fall, but you can fight them by smearing yourself with kerosene. I dread for one of them to bite me, because I know they're full of poison," reported one Alabama woman. "You can't tell Bob anything about them, though. He thinks they don't carry chills; but I know they're bad as moccasins for their size."[88] Other FWP interviews echoed the persistence of nonmosquito theories of malaria causation. In describing health on his former plantation, an old black man explained simply, "But the slaves used to get sick. There was jaundice in them bottoms."[89] A school cafeteria worker who lived with eight children in a three-room house remembered happier days on her father's South Carolina farm. "Them days on the farm was good old days. . . . Once I 'member we had a awful time when we was out there. All the children but one had took the malaria fever and we was in some fix. The water got bad somehow and its a wonder all of us didn't die."[90] Bad water and bad places continued to explain malaria for these rural southerners well into the 1930s. Interviews from the FWP support a broad range of etiological understanding concerning malaria, which was reflected in the physicians' description of the ignorant masses.

Some took malaria lightly as a disease experience, perhaps most particularly when men commented on their wives' affliction with chills. One backwoods misogynist was frank in his discussions with a male interviewer, expressing his opinion that "[a] woman's like a dumb animal—like a cow or a bitch dog. You got to frail 'em with a stick now an' then to make 'em look up to you." He told the story of his common-law wife Nora, who had given him six children in eleven years. After that "she got to whar she weren't wuth keepin'. She got to creepin' 'bout th' house like a wood-legged woman, an' her hide got as yaller as a persimmon. I got thinkin' once that I'd run 'er off—she weren't doin' me no good." He went on to describe the final throes of her mortal illness, without much sympathy. "She was tuk with a chill one night, an she went out a awful way. . . . When she was lyin' thar tremblin' with th' chill, she kep raisin' up her hands an' yellin', 'He's in th' kitchen now! Th' devil's in th' kitchen, an' he's comin' after me.'" In her delirium she was wracked with guilt that she had not been lawfully wed.[91]

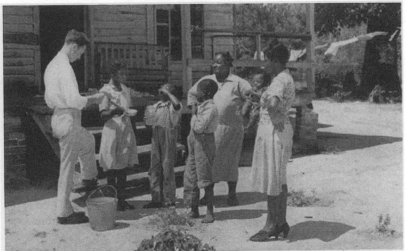

U. S. Public Health Service

**"No Fooling! Take Your Quinine Pills Right Now"**

The doctor takes no chances as he distributes a daily dose to a family near Savannah, Georgia, in a malarial area. Such preventive measures suppress fever symptoms if medicine is taken in early evening. Quinine remains in the blood stream only about 12 hours; the Anopheles mosquito, which carries malaria, generally bites only after dark. This family is urged to sleep in screened rooms, dry up small pools of water, and spray larger breeding places with crude oil.

"No Fooling! Take Your Quinine Pills Right Now!" This USPHS photo illustrates one encounter between the medical and southern rural worldviews around 1920. The white doctor is accompanied by a black assistant, distinctive from the family in her dressy shoes, earrings, and hair styling, whose holding of the baby while the medicine is distributed may have helped smooth a somewhat awkward situation.
(Photographic Collection, Records of the USPHS, Record Group 90, NACP)

A similar attitude emerged from a more humorous tale told by an Alabama country woman.

"I got good and tickled at [Bob, my husband] last year," she said. "Me and Beatrice [her daughter] had been havin' chills, shaking our bones nearly out, and sufferin' with high fevers after they was over. We really needed to have a doctor, or at least some chill tonic, but Bob didn't do a thing about it. He didn't give us an[y] comfort when we was havin' them, and he expected us to be up to cook at meal times."

"Well, it went on like that for a good while, with him not payin' us any mind. Then one day, he come down with a chill. Lawsy me, I never have heard anybody take on so. He shook till the bed like to have fell down, and when the chill was over, he took fever. I was sorry for him as I could be, but I couldn't help bein' tickled; he looked so funny and helpless lyin' up there in bed, groanin' like he was dyin'.

"When I saw how bad he was sufferin', I sent Bea over to fetch Dr. Lawson, and he come quick. He got his fever down, but he told him that another hard chill would strike him the day after the next, and sure enough, one did. But I got tickled again that day, too, because Bob wouldn't budge out of the house; he'd just sit and look at the clock like it was goin' to run off someplace.

"I've heard there's good in ever'thing, and I s'pose there was good in him takin sick. Me or the girls don't start shakin' real good now before he's back with a doctor, and flutterin' around like a chicken with its head cut off. B'lieve me, we made a Christian out of him when he seen how bad a chill was."[92]

It is hard to know what attitude toward malaria's visitations was the common one, but certainly this man learned a new appreciation of what one modern victim of malaria has described as "an icy bite in your marrow," accompanied by a headache that is like "a searing iron in your brain."[93]

Deaths due to malaria undoubtedly caused great grief among family members left behind. The sadness of one black woman in rural North Carolina was painfully evident. "When she was four years old she was tuk wid a fever cake in her side," she said of her daughter, who probably suffered from the splenomegaly of malaria. "At fust it was no bigger'n dis snuff box lid, but it kep' growin', from her navel to her thigh, a great knot in her side. I worked on her wid tar and grease, made her a tar jacket, done anything folks'd tell me." Although she had no access to a physician, family members helped her care for the girl. "When de child died, . . . [I] tuk to grief. . . . I hated to bury my little girl."[94] A Texas man's account of malaria's toll was equally poignant. Initially his family's life together had been good. "We cleared up 'bout thirty acres and had plenty of barn and shed room built fer all de feed we could raise. We lived here till mah chilluns was grown." He went on, sadly, "Mah wife died here wid malaria and chills. She had one chill after another. Her health was good when we first moved here, but 'long 'bout four years befo' she died, her health broke and we spent lots of money for medicine and doctors, but dey didn't do her no good."[95]

Although public health officials tended to see southerners as ignorant and apathetic, the reality was much more complex. The doctors spoke in a language that at times must have been incomprehensible to them, especially in its assumptions about disease classification and causation. For a people who still thought in terms of undifferentiated fevers and chills, and the dangers of bad places, the official talk of hookworm, malaria, pellagra, typhoid, and tuberculosis must have been quite puzzling, not to mention all the steps that must be taken to combat each problem individually. One USPHS photograph (undated) encapsulates the perplexities of that encounter.[96] The USPHS doctor is distributing quinine, probably during one of the 1920s campaigns described in Chapter 4. While the family illustrated no doubt appreciated the free medicine, their faces and stance do not express complete confidence. Most likely the young woman in heels is working with the white doctor, offering a bridge between two worldviews. She appears to be the speaker, urging the family to take quinine and trying to break through their apathy and distrust. The dramatic experience of chills and fever was hard to ignore, but it is difficult in this context to distinguish a patient's apathy ("I don't care") from fatalism ("there is nothing I can do about it"), especially when the patient feared speaking to these men in authority. The clash of worldviews that underlay any attempt at conversation was profound. The population most receptive to the public health message was likely the schoolchildren, who absorbed this strange story about mosquitoes and germs with readiness when their elders found it mysterious and threatening.

# Chapter 7                          Denouement

The 1940s were watershed years for malaria control. After decades of waxing and waning in the rural South, malaria suddenly disappeared. The major drop occurred from about 1938 to 1942, although a few indigenous cases would still be recorded in the late 1940s. Paradoxically, the period of steepest drop did not coincide with the period of greatest public spending on malaria, which actually came after the disease's steep decline. From 1942 to 1950 public health officials at the state and federal level spent more than $50 million to control malaria.[1] Malaria assumed preeminent importance during the war years, both at home and abroad, bringing the malariologist's craft to the forefront of public health work. But why now, after the field had suffered neglect for so many years? And why now, when the disease had almost vanished?

Like most historical phenomena, the causes were multifactorial. First, malaria cases and deaths were so inaccurately reported that malariologists were fooled about the prevalence of the disease. They also saw it as a disease of mysterious cycles and feared that the low point of the early 1940s was to be followed by a later resurgence. This fear was supplemented by concern that after the Second World War, parasite-infested soldiers returning to the United States from malarious areas of the world would start new outbreaks. So a certain panic underlay the calls for attention to this problem. Second, malaria was *the* disease of World War II—it had a massive impact on the war effort abroad, and the crisis climate spread to the American South. Military metaphors targeted malaria as an enemy and its eradication as "winning the war," helping to create the passion to wipe out the enemy at home and prevent the invasion of the foreigner in the bodies of returning GIs. Third, malaria became the basis of institution building for the public health arm of the federal government. The Centers for Disease Control (CDC) grew directly out of the malaria control effort, so its founders had a large stake in the promotion of malaria eradication. Finally, the technological innovation of DDT offered a new, powerful, economical weapon. Malaria could be eradicated once and for all, easily, without addressing the problem of poverty, which so vexed other public health questions. The public demand for DDT did much to solidify the image and reputation of the fledgling CDC.[2]

Yet this burst of activity occurred when malaria seemed to be disappearing, a recent development that took malariologists quite by surprise. During the 1930s malaria rates had shot up to levels not seen since the very early years of the century—just at a time when slim public health budgets discouraged efforts towards surveillance and control.[3] Certainly, in 1942, a few significant pockets of infection remained in the South. State and federal officials conducted early trials of spraying DDT in the shacks bordering the Santee-Cooper Reservoir of coastal South Carolina and the swampy lowlands of western Tennessee, because there measurable malaria still existed.[4] But such spots were shrinking and fading. A USPHS team noted with amazement in 1950 that they had to go back to 1942 to find cases of locally transmitted malaria.[5] Already in 1940 cases were so unusual in the New Orleans Charity Hospital that a malaria patient was a rare discovery, suitable for wide display to medical students.[6]

Contemporary malariologists were not blind to the decline in malaria; they saw it, but they feared that the disease could revive at any time. Since they had no clear understanding of why malaria was disappearing, it could certainly just as mysteriously reverse its course. Faust and others frequently argued that malaria in the United States was a disease of cycles, and by the early 1940s the South was overdue for its latest peak. The federal agency that was created to fight malaria in 1942 even put the graph of malaria's twentieth-century peaks and troughs on its cover, to emphasize the likelihood of a new upsurge.[7] Malariologists also worried about the reliability of their data that showed low malaria rates.

The problems linked to the mass movement of men at war added considerably to this anxiety. During World War II millions of soldiers passed through the training camps of the South. Many domestic cases of malaria had weakened soldiers traveling the same course in World War I; federal and state officials were determined that the World War II soldier remain "fit to fight" and not be stricken low by the South's endemic disease of enervation.[8] As the war went on, and more and more troops returned from malarious areas, concern shifted to the problem of men bringing the infection back with them and starting new epidemics in disease-free areas.[9] Malariologists warned that the disease promised to be "a lively corpse" whose possible resurgence should not be dismissed.[10] If their concern in retrospect seems overblown, it is hard to be too condemnatory. The same could be said of the swine influenza affair of the mid-1970s—epidemiologists made their best guess about how disease cycles were going to happen and preferred preventing a major outbreak to treating the cases afterward.[11]

Another factor in building the federal and state response was the prominence that malaria acquired during the war. Multiple documents cited it as "the #1 disease of World War II"—as it certainly was in the Pacific theater and to a lesser extent in Africa and Italy. Malaria was a major factor in the fall of Bataan and in other early war disasters. It put many more men in the hospital than battle casualties, in ratios at times as high as 30 to 1. General MacArthur told malariologist Paul Russell that "it would be a very long war indeed if for every division facing the Japanese he must count on a second division in hospital with acute malaria, and a third division in a convalescent depot with relapsing malaria."[12] This early experience with malaria received much publicity, and the government's massive response became central to the war effort.[13] Because of a quinine shortage (Japan monopolized the supply), pharmacologists quickly found new drugs to take its place. Army researchers combined the best available insecticide, pyrethrum, with freon to create the first insect bomb. Troops were bombarded with an educational campaign to teach them to avoid malaria. And in the last two years of the war, DDT was used to make the Pacific safe for democracy.[14]

Malaria was big news, and its eradication was discussed with all the jingoism of wartime. Further, since it was such an important disease abroad, it must be an important disease at home too. A new malaria awareness resulted from the war, as well as a new awareness of its malignity.[15] One army physician described this change in a popular science article published in 1946, arguing, "Malaria has always been a scourge of the world, but not until the recent global war has its devastations been brought forcefully to the attention of the people of this country."[16] Protecting American troops at home, and workers at militarily important industrial sites, became a dominant war objective, covered in patriotic gloss and fervor. As one navy physician said, "To minimize the threat of malaria is to jeopardize the war effort."[17] To relax would have been traitorous. The U.S. Army distributed a training film about malaria that illustrated this new urgency, labeling the anopheles mosquito "Public Enemy #1" and calling on all Americans to fight this grave pestilence.[18]

The first money spent was on the areas around military sites and important factories. The Malaria Control in War Areas agency (MCWA), set up in 1942 as a wing of the U.S. Public Health Service, had as its specific objective the creation of one-mile safe zones around these military sites, of which there were many in the South. A cartoon from 1943 illustrated MCWA's role as a barrier between the infected mosquito carrying the bomb of malaria, and valued locales such as troop camps, ships, and industries.[19] MCWA cooperated with state boards of health on a program of temporary, immediately effective control measures, especially spreading anopheles breeding sites with oil or arsenic compounds.[20] It also funded research laboratories and had side interests in typhus and yellow fever control. The federal and state governments combined spent nearly $25 million on domestic malaria prevention during the war years. By 1945 MCWA had more than four thousand employees.[21]

As the war went on, the focus of MCWA shifted 180 degrees. Where once it had targeted civilians with malaria as the danger and soldiers as the victims, by 1944 it was targeting returning GIs bringing the disease home to potentially infectible areas.[22] As evidence of malaria's new rareness in the South emerged, malariologists became anxious to preserve this potentially tenuous state of affairs. MCWA researchers determined that foreign malarial plasmodia were easily transmitted by domestic mosquitoes. There would be no natural barrier to the transmission.[23]

Indeed, in 1944 when Congress debated a bill to reorganize the USPHS by consolidating prior laws, codifying personnel promotion, salary, and benefit issues, and specifically listing its multiple duties, the threat of malaria from returning servicemen was invoked as an imminent peril that justified the measure. As Senator Elbert Thomas of Utah noted, the bill "does not add to the law of the land . . . but merely brings the law up to date, in such a way that one of the most vital and most necessary agencies of our Government may operate unhampered, at a time when our country is really imperiled." He went on to list two such dangers—tuberculosis, and the fact that "there are coming back to our country from all parts of the world men afflicted with malaria and other sicknesses." The bill passed the 78th Congress, and became Public Law 410.[24]

This shift in focus reinforced the fact that MCWA personnel never claimed to be *controlling* malaria. Rather, they were *preventing* it. They measured the abundance of anopheles mosquitoes in their protection zones, not the presence of malaria cases. In fact, there were almost no malaria cases to discuss in their zones.[25] The change in emphasis from controlling malaria to minimizing mosquitoes was especially evident in the maps drawn by malaria field-workers during the late 1930s and 1940s. During the late 1930s, when communities in eastern North Carolina had been mapped, each house was labeled by occupant name, and the number of malaria cases found there was noted. The MCWA maps from the mid-1940s, on the other hand, concentrated on the areas around militarily important sites and are entirely concerned with indicating mosquito densities at the various "trapping stations" set up to monitor the mosquito population. In their reports, malaria case data is replaced with mosquito counts.[26]

This lack of attention to actual malaria did not go unnoted at the time. Stanley Freeborn, a senior USPHS physician, commented aptly in 1944, "I think some of us who are closest to the work sometimes confuse costs, size of projects, gallons of oil and mosquito densities as criteria of accomplishment." After admitting that "our only true measure is the presence,

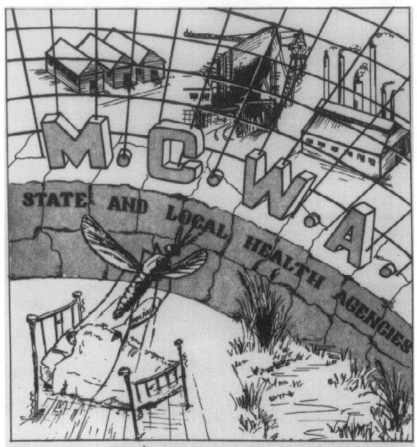

M.C.W.A. IS THE SUPERSTRUCTURE BUILT UPON THE SOLID FOUNDATION OF STATE AND LOCAL HEALTH AGENCIES FOR THE PROTECTION OF FIGHTING MEN AND WAR WORKERS.

M.C.W.A. The goal of the MCWA was to maintain a malaria-free zone around war industries and encampments. This function is illustrated here with a stone wall and mesh fence that keeps the mosquito, carrying a malaria bomb, from traveling to barracks, a ship-building site, or a factory.
(*Malaria Control in War Areas, 1942–1943*, 5)

severity, reduction or absence of malaria," he was unsure whether to take credit for the lack of malaria in the protected areas.[27] Still, he and other senior MCWA and military public health officials were proud of the fact that the domestic military malaria rate was so low in World War II compared to World War I. But the paucity of malaria cases was not seen as an indication for them to shut up shop and go home. The threat was still there, and the low prevalence of the disease was a sign of their success, not their superfluousness. The MCWA reports emphasized how much work had been accomplished, and the U.S. Congress rewarded them with increased funding each year.[28]

Malaria field-workers also had doubts about this switch to counting mosquitoes instead of malaria, but the officials at MCWA were impervious to criticism of their decision. For example, in 1944 sanitary engineer John Porter of New Orleans responded to a MCWA field bulletin (April 1944) with indignation. MCWA had set as a standard of "adequate *anopheles* control" the count of ten or fewer mosquitoes at a measurement station over a twenty-four-hour period. When certain areas under the engineer's supervision were designated as "out of control," he countered angrily that the figures were arbitrary and had nothing to do with the truly important measure, the community's malaria morbidity. "If effectiveness of malaria control is to be based solely on any arbitrary number of Anopheles Q. mosquitoes found in 'A' stations, then the designation of MCWA is a misnomer," Porter claimed. "It is illogical to take as a criterion of effectiveness of malaria control any arbitrary figure for station counts. . . . It should be remembered that *mosquito control* is a means to an end and not the end (objective) in itself."[29]

George Bradley, MCWA's senior entomologist, responded to Porter's letter with an answer that mainly defended the count of ten anopheles per day as the appropriate measure of dangerous mosquito density. When he addressed the crucial choice of MCWA to focus on mosquitoes and not malaria, he did so by rather circular means. "The control measures being prosecuted on the M.C.W.A. program are almost entirely directed toward reducing the number of adult anophelines by larvicidal measures," he admitted. "I fail to see where it is illogical to determine the results of this work by the reduction brought about in the density of these mosquitoes," he concluded. He then went on to say that, yes, it would be more satisfying to measure the actual malaria rate. But this is not possible, so "the only way that the effect of our work in decreasing the potential malaria hazard can be determined is by measuring the decreased densities of anophelines." Once he had redefined MCWA's role as preventing rather than controlling malaria, he was on firm logical ground in counting mosquitoes. But MCWA's second name was control, and no senior MCWA official ever directly addressed the fallacy of controlling an absent disease.[30]

MCWA planners seemed to know that counting mosquitoes was a second-best strategy for gauging malaria control, but that they had neither the time nor the ability to base the campaign on blood smear prevalence data. Late in 1942, an internal memorandum from MCWA statistician Elliott Pennell to his boss summarized these problems. Even after vast numbers of smears had been taken, he despaired of deriving accurate indices of malaria's prevalence from them. He cited problems of local technical skill, inappropriate study site locations, the backlog of microscopic examinations once the slides were obtained, and poor record keeping on the local level. MCWA needed rapidly to mobilize a malaria control program, and relying on blood smears for monitoring success promised to be too slow and inadequate.[31] Instead, MCWA's leaders chose to follow the mosquito census.

MCWA never discussed any strategy other than mosquito control as a method of limiting malaria in the United States. Even in 1945, it rejected out of hand the opportunity to test atabrine, and later chloroquine, on the malarious population around the Santee-Cooper Reservoir. The use of these medications, MCWA believed, would interfere with the parasitemia reservoir (i.e., the sick bodies) and thus destroy the data to be found from mosquito dissections. By this time American malariologists were almost entirely "mosquito-focused," and the possibility of attacking malaria in any other way was remote from their minds.

In 1944 MCWA's head, Dr. L. L. Williams, used the threat of the returning GI to call for an all-out eradication campaign for malaria. The agency was already in place—MCWA—and the tools were. He saw eradication as the ultimate solution to the imported malaria problem.[32] In early 1945 Congress voted funds to extend the MCWA program in the ways Williams outlined, and the eradication campaign was on.[33] The MCWA "extended program" was renamed the Communicable Disease Center in that year.[34] (The CDC kept its initials but changed its name in later years.)

In retrospect, the imported disease threat seems to have been minor, but in 1944–45 it looked very real.[35] As late as 1952, the CDC's Justin Andrews stated at a staff meeting that "this country was now free of malaria but we must keep it that way." The minutes then recorded, "He pointed out that no one knows why malaria has decreased so greatly. Certainly there are some influences which are yet unknown and which are not connected with Malaria Control programs." Andrews went on to say that "no one knows why the returning soldiers from World War II, many of whom have recurrent malaria, and the present group of soldiers from Korea do not spark an outbreak of malaria."[36] Malariologists at the USPHS may have used malaria control as a foundation for institution building, but there is no indication that they did so with deliberate deceit.[37] Yes, by 1945, malaria was at the lowest level ever recorded, but that only meant an opportunity for "striking while the iron is hot," not cause for complacency.[38] On the other hand, an agency was in place with those thousands of employees; that size must have created a sort of inertia effect for continuance.[39]

The final factor in the large commitment to malaria eradication during the 1940s was the advent of a new piece of technology—DDT (dichloro-diphenyl-trichloro-ethane). Paul Mueller, a Swiss chemist working for Geigy, first identified the insecticidal properties of DDT in 1939, while looking for a good compound to kill moths in clothing. Switzerland was neutral, and Geigy offered the compound to both Germany and the United States. In America it was added to a pile of compounds that were being actively tested for insecticidal properties by the Department of Agriculture laboratory in Orlando.[40] Just as a quinine shortage in the war had led to a big research effort for new drugs, a pyrethrum shortage led to a search for other insecticides to take its place.[41] DDT was one of many compounds explored, and it was its ability to kill lice that first earned it attention. As it was tested on other insects, the excitement about its potential grew exponentially. DDT not only killed insects immediately, it continued killing for up to three months.[42] American personnel first tested its field use in liberated Naples, where spraying the entire population stopped a typhus epidemic—a monumental achievement under wartime conditions.[43] As an editorial in the *American Journal of Public Health* noted in 1946, "the use of DDT has worked a scientific miracle in the control of typhus fever," preventing what would have been "one of the great typhus epidemics."[44] DDT was also used in the Pacific theater, where whole islands were sprayed by air to prepare for the safe forward movement of American troops.[45]

DDT was called "the atomic bomb of the insect world"; the 1945 MCWA report even showed the mushroom cloud on its cover to emphasize the connection.[46] The first head of the CDC pointed out that from the standpoint of insect control technology, World War II was a huge success. "It liberated DDT from oblivion, to fulfill its glorious destiny."[47] Popular literature referred to it as "the wonder insecticide of World War II."[48] It was a great scientific discovery that had won the war and demonstrated American scientific prowess. When the malariologists at the CDC decided to build their malaria eradication program around the use of DDT, they built on all this public fervor.[49]

The American people wanted DDT. Rarely has a public health effort had such a strong public demand. The desire was to kill not just mosquitoes but flies, bedbugs, lice, fleas, and cockroaches. Although knowledge about DDT's toxicity was already accumulating, and people were warned to avoid skin contact, the toxicity message was lost amid the glorification of this new wonder chemical.[50] MCWA did its part to promote the chemical, for as its annual report noted in 1945, the "wholesale spraying of the interiors of half a million homes in a free country poses certain problems in public relations."[51] By and large the message traveled faster than the spray crews. People in nontargeted areas were angry at being left out. Only 2 percent of householders refused the first year's spraying in 1945 overall; in North Carolina the spray crews found 10 percent resistance on the first round, but as the news spread about DDT's wondrous effects, less than 1 percent shut them out on the second round.[52] People were "pawing at the ground with eagerness," according to one popular press article.[53] This eagerness helped the MCWA effort enormously, because prior preparation and cooperation by householders markedly reduced the cost of spraying.

The MCWA (and then the newly christened CDC) plan for DDT use in malaria eradication was simple in concept. The first step was to identify counties with more than five malaria cases per 100,000 population during 1938–42, which qualified them as officially malarious. Next, with cooperation of state public health units, spray crews were sent to these counties to spray all house and privy walls with DDT every three months for the duration of the mosquito season. The effectiveness of the program was to be monitored by counting the number of live anopheles mosquitoes found in the houses at given intervals after the spray crews' departure. This measure was based on the assumption that mosquitoes invading houses would routinely be killed by resting on DDT-coated walls, ineluctably breaking the chain of transmission from malaria case to malaria case. In its first year the program reached over half a million Southern homes. These numbers escalated to more than a million a year in the late 1940s.[54]

In 1947 the original two-year extended program was expanded to a five-year (1947–52) eradication campaign. It built on the strength of DDT as a technology and the postwar fear of malaria. Finishing the fight was the patriotic thing to do.[55] As the army's chief medical spokesman proclaimed, "[W]e must not demobilize until we have defeated our enemies."[56] It was easy to see how malaria would be controlled by the mass death of mosquitoes, and it was relatively cheap.[57] Compared to prior technologies, DDT killed mosquitoes for a fraction of the cost. Each house could be sprayed, and thus effectively mosquito-proofed, for only seventy-four cents, according to one estimate. From 1947 to 1950 the CDC directed the spraying of nearly five million homes in the South; by 1950 only nineteen indigenous malaria cases could be located.[58] The spraying program was called off in 1951, as malaria had apparently been eradicated.

The malariologists guiding the activities of the extended MCWA program (1945–47) and then the CDC's malaria eradication program (1947–52) knew that very little malaria was left in the South. They never tried to justify their programs in terms of dropping malaria rates but in the reduction of mosquito density. Justin Andrews, head of the CDC, was explicit in his focus on heavy anopheles breeding areas, rather than sites of known disease.[59] The measurable goal was to kill mosquitoes, not to decrease malaria cases. He was acutely aware that even the apparent drop in malaria mortality from 1946 to 1947 was almost entirely due to a change in reporting requirements rather than in an actual change in disease rate, and he honestly admitted it. Still, he feared the lurking disease, the closeted demon ready to strike should economic disaster return to the South. No one yet knew why malaria had receded; hence there was great concern that it might come back. As a USPHS spokesman said in 1949, "The possibility of renewed transmission cannot be overlooked as long as the reasons for the recession of malaria are not understood completely."[60] In retrospect Andrews justified the expenditure on the DDT program by noting that in 1946 the confusion about prevalence of malaria persisted, there was great fear of a cycle peak, and the returning GI bringing malaria haunted malariologists.[61]

Retrospective analyses by Andrews, Paul Russell, and Alexander Langmuir, all men at the center of the malaria wars of the 1940s, were murky on the overall effect of the massive DDT spraying program. Russell claimed that it probably interrupted a "prolonged condition of light endemicity," while Andrews wondered if it did even that much.[62] Langmuir wrote Andrews, "Even in this country [the United States], it is wholly impossible to judge the extent to which the control of malaria is related to organized insect control." After citing Andrews's own work, he went on, "I certainly concur with your conclusion that the decline in malaria in this country had started well before the DDT period, and the best we can claim in this country is that we 'kicked a dying dog.'"[63] Two early pilot projects that actually tried to correlate malaria rates with DDT use, in South Carolina (in the Santee-Cooper Reservoir area) and Puerto Rico, failed to show a significant difference between treated and untreated areas.[64] These marginal results were dismissed by those who felt drawn to DDT as the atomic bomb of insecticides, whose power to destroy mosquitoes, and hence malaria, seemed self-evident.

The CDC's spokespersons were not shy about touting the importance of World War II in increasing the budgets of the USPHS and its components. An orientation manual for new CDC employees noted that the war brought the service "the responsibility for administering unprecedented sums." In 1946 this budget reached its peak of more than $136 million (compared to the 1939 budget of $25 million). While it dropped to $104 million in 1947, the appropriation was back up to $118 million in 1948. The CDC put the bulk of its share into the DDT program, although by the end of the 1940s its directors were turning to other infectious diseases, and to the concept of surveillance for lightly present but threatening diseases, as a way to justify continued budgetary appropriations. After the war, the budget for malaria control was continually cut, but the CDC put its principal focus on the DDT campaign (in concert with the state boards of health) and denied funding to research areas that looked at other questions in malaria control.[65]

The most significant effect of the malaria eradication campaign was to build the CDC into a permanent agency for tracking, preventing, and controlling domestic infectious diseases. That accomplishment was constructed out of the "successful" war on malaria, however unimpressive that "success" may seem in hindsight. Building on the military metaphors of the time and the glamour of DDT, the malaria campaigners led federal and state governments deeper into preventive medicine and justified the creation of an important institution for investigating and fighting other infectious diseases. Perhaps this was worth the $50 million spent, even if its effect on malaria prevalence was ultimately hard to measure.

## Epilogue

However it had happened, indigenous malaria was gone from the United States. Over the next half century cases of malaria would reappear, to be sure, but almost all would be traceable to infections acquired in other countries. American troops brought malaria home from Korea, Vietnam, and Somalia, although concerted military efforts kept the disease from spreading to civilians. In 1979 a flood of refugees from Southeast Asia carried malaria parasites to the United States, causing a brief flurry of public health excitement before the CDC contained the cases. The surveillance instituted by the CDC in the late 1940s, perhaps the greatest legacy of the MCWA program, has continued to the present day. Malaria is a reportable disease, and few cases escape the CDC's awareness. There have been a few indigenous cases in the past few years, cases that cannot be attributed to foreign travel or known contacts with malarious persons, but by and large it is safe to say that malaria as a significant threat to the nation's health has left the United States for good.[66]

This story is in sharp contrast to events elsewhere in the world. While malaria was vanquished from most developed countries after World War II, it remained (and remains) a major problem for those underdeveloped parts of the globe that are tropical enough to host anopheles and its parasitic companion. Given the apparent success of DDT in eradicating malaria in North America, Europe, and elsewhere, in 1955 the World Health Organization (WHO) launched a worldwide campaign to destroy malaria. Meeting in Mexico City, WHO delegates responded not only to arguments about the importance of malaria as a global killer, but also to early reports that some insects were becoming resistant to the insecticide. The time was ripe for a massive campaign to wipe out anopheles mosquitoes before invulnerable generations had time to evolve. The plan called for all shelters (huts, houses, barns) to be sprayed with DDT, up to four times a year if necessary. Spraying was to continue until surveillance showed an absence of malarial parasites in the blood of area residents.[67]

A prominent American malariologist, Paul Russell of the Rockefeller Foundation, was key in shaping the WHO's plan. After outlining the rationale for the eradication campaign, he drew explicitly on the American case, among others, for evidence that such efforts could be successful. "In 1951 it began to be apparent that certain Anopheles vector species were becoming resistant to DDT and others to BHC [benzene hexachloride] and dieldrin," Russell began. "This appearance of resistance suggested that the indefinite continuance of a residual spraying campaign under the concept of malaria control might become impossible," so it was necessary to switch from a concept of control (or minimization) to complete eradication. He called on history to demonstrate that eradication was possible. "This point of view was emphasized when it became apparent during 1954 that malaria had been eradicated by residual spraying from wide areas of the United States, Puerto Rico, Venezuela, British Guiana, Italy, and elsewhere," Russell argued. "So, it was both a logical and a progressive move, when in October 1954 the representatives of 21 American countries in the XIVth Pan-American Sanitary Conference in Santiago, Chile, approved a programme calling for nothing less than the eradication of malaria from the Americas." Further, it made complete sense that "[t]he World Health Organization in Mexico City in May 1955 at its VIIIth World Health Assembly adopted malaria eradication as the goal of its antimalaria activities."[68] Russell had his doubts that DDT was completely responsible for the disappearance of malaria from the United States, but he was certain that it offered the world's best hope for the disease's conquest.

The WHO program got off to an energetic start, but even from the beginning it was flawed. No one ever seriously thought the deep and complex presence of malaria in Africa could be conquered, although there was hope for control and reduction. There simply was not enough money or political will to effect a thorough program to attack all pockets of residual disease ready to rekindle a malaria epidemic. This was true elsewhere as well. The DDT campaign did cause a significant reduction in malaria morbidity and mortality, but as the 1960s progressed it became obvious that it was ultimately failing in its goal of eradication. More and more mosquitoes developed pesticide resistance; the pesticides themselves came to be seen as more and more toxic, and more and more parasites developed resistance to available drugs. The parasite was winning, and in 1969 the WHO declared defeat.[69]

Since the 1970s malaria has come back from its temporary deflation at the hands of WHO eradicators. Areas once free of the disease are now seeing rising numbers of cases. No new control strategy has emerged in recent years to replace the faulty DDT spraying plan. Affluent Americans traveling to malarious areas can easily protect their health by taking any of several effective drugs, although they may not appreciate the concomitant side effects. But these medications are too costly for most of the third world's inhabitants. In the last two decades researchers have tried to invent a malaria vaccine, with limited success. Newer insecticides are, if anything, even more toxic to the environment than DDT. Malariologists in developing countries are turning increasingly to low-technology solutions such as insecticide-soaked bednets, as nothing else is available.[70]

Does the history of malaria's conquest in the United States offer any clues for malariologists seeking to control the disease in tropical countries? In America malaria thrived where impoverished, malnourished people lived in porous housing near anopheles breeding grounds, and they contracted a disease for which they could not, by and large, acquire effective medication for suppression or cure. Rising prosperity played a role in supplying better housing, quinine, and adequate food, but this did not effect the last holdouts of malaria in the rural South in the late 1930s. The critical change was the movement of the at-risk population away from the mosquito, breaking the tenuous chain of malaria transmission. The major DDT spraying program of the 1940s finished off what pockets of disease remained. Facilitating a similar population translocation in the hyperendemic areas of Africa and Asia is neither feasible or desirable. It is hard to know whether the American DDT spraying campaign would have been successful without it.

A further issue that clouds any comparison of the American case with developing countries, especially in Africa, concerns congenital immunities to malaria. Absence of the Duffy antigen offers almost complete protection against *vivax* malaria, but it is *falciparum* that is the major problem in Africa and South Asia. But those traits, such as abnormal hemoglobins, that protect the bearer against death from *falciparum* malaria at the same time make him or her a tolerant carrier of the parasite. Anywhere such traits abound, malaria will be all the more difficult to eradicate. In the United States these traits cluster in African-Americans; where the proportion of African-Americans was highest, such as in the Carolina lowlands and the Mississippi Delta, malaria was at its most severe. Still, the most malarious areas of the American South would not approach the census of excellent adult malaria carriers present in the hyperendemic areas of Africa and Asia.

In general, the malaria problem in the United States never approached that of tropical developing countries in severity. The anopheles mosquitoes resident in the United States, *maculipennis* and *quadrimaculatus,* are weak vectors compared with those of Africa and Asia, especially *Anopheles gambiae.* The American mosquitoes are less efficient at picking up and depositing parasites. Although adequate to do the job, they do not do it well, and they have fewer months of the year in which to do it.

Altogether, comparisons of the American success story with the African and Asian failure sagas illustrate mainly that malaria is easier to eradicate where it is less entrenched. It is easier to eradicate where the population as a whole is prosperous, and the federal government has ample funds to apply available technology thoroughly. It is hard to imagine malaria returning in any significant degree to the United States. Most of its inhabitants live in screened dwellings, with at least emergency room access to medical care in case of significant illness. CDC surveillance of malaria means that any local outbreak will be quenched before it extends beyond a few cases. Short of a major societal upheaval in the wake of natural or man-made devastation, malaria will probably never again be a major public health problem in the United States. It has become one of the diseases of the American past, such as polio, yellow fever, cholera, and smallpox, whose disappearance has helped define and create the standard of living expected in the modern, developed world.

Although I have emphasized the role of socioeconomic, geographic, and population movement in limiting malaria in the United States, it would be inaccurate to close without some final tribute to the men and women whose deliberate efforts toward malaria control contributed to its disappearance. Paul Russell, writing near the end of his career in 1968, argued: "The present freedom of the United States from malaria is due to many factors but certainly, in no small measure, it stems from those years of active cooperation between the Public Health Service, state and county health departments, and the Rockefeller Foundation, all of which linked resources of men and money in malaria research and training and organization." Russell crowed, "Now, after four centuries of endemicity, malaria has been eradicated from the United States," a "great achievement" for which the country's malariologists deserved great applause.[71] He concluded, "Nothing in the history of public health, it seems to me, equals in determination, accomplishment, and generosity, the performance of the United States in its fight against malaria at home and abroad."[72]

My account varies from Russell's in attributing far more to socioeconomic forces and far less to deliberate public health activity in the story of malaria's disappearance. But is hard not to have sympathy for and pride in the men and women who tramped through swamps, stared all day long through microscopes, and otherwise risked comfort and health to bring malaria under control in the American South. The history of malaria during the twentieth century is one of triumphal success in developed countries and overwhelming failure in tropical developing ones. It is all too unfortunate that the reasons for this variance lie not in science and technology, of which we have a rich supply, but rather in the social, economic, and political forces over which the public health community ultimately has little control. Paul Russell perhaps put it best: "What a paradox! Man, with his incredible machines and his streamlined science, stricken each year in millions because he fails to outwit a mosquito carrying Death in its spittle!"[73]

# Notes

ARCHIVE ABBREVIATIONS

FWP-SHC:  Federal Writers' Project Papers. Southern Historical Collection. University of
North Carolina at Chapel Hill. Chapel Hill, North Carolina.

RAC:  Rockefeller Archive Center. North Tarrytown, New York.

NACP:  National Archives. College Park, Maryland.

CDCA:  Centers for Disease Control Archives. National Archives Southeast. East
Point, Georgia.

INTRODUCTION

1.  "Malaria: Reduced to the Vanishing Point," *Public Health Rep* 65 (1950): 1689;
C. P. Stevick, "Has Malaria Disappeared?" *N C Med J* 12 (1951): 438–40.

2.  Stanley C. Oaks, Jr., et al., eds., *Malaria: Obstacles and Opportunities. A
Report of the Committee for the Study on Malaria Prevention and Control: Status Review and Alternative Strategies, Division of International Health* (Washington: National Academy Press, 1991), 1.

3.  See, for example, J. Sunstrom et al., "Mosquito-Transmitted Malaria—Michigan, 1995," *Morb Mort Wkly Rep* 45 (1996): 398–400; M. Dawson et al., "Prob-
able Locally Acquired Mosquito-Transmitted *Plasmodium vivax* Infection—
Georgia, 1996," *Morb Mort Wkly Rep* 46 (1997): 264–67; C. del Rio et al.,
"Malaria in an Immigrant and Travelers—Georgia, Vermont, and Tennessee,
1996," *Morb Mort Wkly Rep* 46 (1997): 536–39. Two cases acquired in Florida
made headlines in August 1996: "Officials Look for Source of Last Month's
Malaria Cases in Florida," *News Observer (Raleigh, N.C.)*, Aug. 5, 1996, 5A.
Two more indigenous cases were discovered on Long Island in 1999. John T.
McQuiston, "Officials Try to Find Origin of Malaria in L. I. Boys," *New York
Times,* Sept. 2, 1999, B5.

4.  Robertson Davies, *The Deptford Trilogy* (1970, 1972, and 1975; reprint New
York: Viking Penguin, 1983).

5.  The best history of competing schools of malaria control is Socrates Litsios,
*The Tomorrow of Malaria* (Wellington, New Zealand: Pacific Press, 1996). Litsios carries his account through the failed WHO effort of 1955–69 and
beyond, showing the value of history for understanding where the WHO went
wrong.

6. Margaret Humphreys, *Yellow Fever and the South* (1992; reprint Baltimore: Johns Hopkins University Press, 1998).

7. Peter Matthiessen, *At Play in the Fields of the Lord* (1965; reprint New York: Bantam Books, 1976), 222, 224.

CHAPTER ONE: THE PESTILENCE THAT STALKS IN DARKNESS

1. Psalms. 91.5–6 Revised Standard Version

2. This information, and that in the following paragraphs, is widely available in tropical medicine textbooks. See, for example, Stephen C. Reed and Carlos C. Campbell, "Malaria," in Paul D. Hoeprich et al., eds., *Infectious Diseases* (Philadelphia: J. B. Lippincott, 1994): 1335–44; W. H. Wernsdorfer and I. McGregor, eds., *Malaria: Principles and Practice of Malariology* (Edinburgh: Churchill Livingstone, 1988); and Donald J. Krogstad, "Plasmodium Species (Malaria)," in Gerald L. Mandel et al., eds., *Principles and Practice of Infectious Disease*, 4th ed. (New York: Churchill Livingstone, 1998): 2415–27.

3. James Stevens Simmons, "The Transmission of Malaria by the Anopheles Mosquitoes of North America," in Forest Ray Moulton, ed., *A Symposium on Human Malaria with Special Reference to North America and the Caribbean Region* (Washington, D.C.: American Association for the Advancement of Science, 1941), 113–30.

4. M. Bruin Mitzmain, "The Malarial Parasite in the Mosquito: The Effects of Low Temperature and Other Factors in its Development," *Public Health Rep* 32 (1917): 1400–13; and G. H. Bradley and W. V. King, "Bionomics and Ecology of Nearctic Anopheles," in Moulton, ed., *Symposium on Human Malaria*, 79–87.

5. John A. Ferrell, "Challenge of Malaria in the South," *Am J Public Health* 21 (1931): 355–74, at 365.

6. Ernest Carroll Faust, "Clinical and Public Health Aspects of Malaria in the United States from an Historical Perspective," *Am J Trop Med* 25 (1945): 185–201, at 190.

7. Menno Jan Bouma and Christopher Dye, "Cycles of Malaria Associated with El Niño in Venezuela," *J Am Med Assoc* 278 (1997): 1772–74.

8. Jeffrey D. Palmer, "Green Ancestry of Malarial Parasites?" *Curr Biol* 2 (1992): 318–20; L. J. Bruce-Chwatt, "Pathogenesis and Paleoepidemiology of Primate Malaria," *Bull World Health Organ* 32 (1965): 363–87; and G. R. Coatney et al., *The Primate Malarias* (Washington, D.C.: Department of Health, Education, and Welfare, 1971).

9. On the evolution and age of plasmodia species, see L. J. Bruce-Chwatt, "History of Malaria from Prehistory to Eradication," in Wernsdorfer and McGregor, eds., *Malaria*, 1–59.

10. Christopher Wills, *Yellow Fever, Black Goddess: The Coevolution of People and Plagues* (Reading, Mass.: Addison-Wesley, 1996).

11. Paul Ewald, *Evolution of Infectious Disease* (Oxford: Oxford University Press, 1994). A recent discussion of *falciparum's* evolution is F. J. Ayala, A. A. Escalante, and S. M. Rich, "Evolution of *Plasmodium* and the Recent

Origin of the World Populations of *Plasmodium falciparum*" *Parassitologia* 41 (1999): 55–68.

12. Frank B. Livingstone, "On the Nonexistence of Human Races," in Sandra Harding, ed., *The "Racial" Economy of Science: Toward a Democratic Future* (Bloomington: Indiana University Press, 1993), 133–41; Nancy Krieger and Mary Bassett, "The Health of Black Folk: Disease, Class, and Ideology in Science," in ibid., 161–69; Nancy Leys Stepan and Sander L. Gilman, "Appropriating the Idioms of Science: The Rejection of Scientific Racism," in ibid., 170–93; and F. James Davis, *Who Is Black? One Nation's Definition* (University Park: Pennsylvania State University Press, 1991).

13. William W. Stead et al., "Racial Differences in Susceptibility to Infection by *Mycobacterium tuberculosis,*" *N Engl J Med* 322 (1990): 422–27; and H. P. Dunstan, "Does Keloid Pathogenesis Hold the Key to Understanding Black/White Differences in Hypertension Severity?" *Hypertension* 26 (1995): 858–62.

14. See, for example, Richard J. David and James W. Collins, Jr., "Differing Birth Weight among Infants of U.S.-born Blacks, African-born Blacks, and U.S.-born Whites," *N Engl J Med* 337 (1997): 1209–14; Mark D. Shriver, "Ethnic Variation as a Key to the Biology of Human Disease," *Ann Intern Med* 127 (1997): 401–03; and D. R. Williams, R. Lavizzo-Mourey, and R. C. Warren, "The Concept of Race and Health Status in America," *Public Health Rep* 109 (1994): 26–41. On the history of the birth weight controversy, see Richard Meckel, "Racialism and Infant Death: Late Nineteenth- and Early Twentieth-century Sociomedical Discourses on African American Infant Mortality," in Lara Marks and Michael Worboys, eds., *Migrants, Minorities and Health: Historical and Contemporary Studies* (London: Routledge, 1997): 70–92.

15. Richard Cooper, "A Note on the Biologic Concept of Race and Its Application in Epidemiological Research," *Am Heart J* 108 (1984): 715–23.

16. Marion Torchia, "Tuberculosis among American Negroes: Medical Research on a Racial Disease, 1830–1959," *J Hist Med Allied Sci* 32 (1977): 252–79.

17. James Jones, *Bad Blood: The Tuskegee Syphilis Experiment* (New York: Free Press, 1981; rev. 1993); and Allan M. Brandt, "Racism and Research: The Case of the Tuskegee Syphilis Study," *Hastings Cent Rep* 8 (1978): 21–29.

18. Julius Chambers, cited in Elizabeth Wellington, "NCCU Breaking Mold—At a Price," *News Observer* (Raleigh, N.C.), Oct. 14, 1997, 1A, 8A.

19. Carlos M. Ferrario, M.D., described the Wake Forest Hypertension Center and its outreach to and research on African-Americans with high blood pressure in his Martin Luther King Memorial Lecture, "Facts, Myths and Treatment of Hypertension in African Americans," presented at Duke University, Jan. 16, 1998; see also Richard Allen Williams, ed., *Textbook of Black-Related Diseases* (New York: McGraw-Hill, 1975). Wake Forest School of Medicine was known as Bowman-Gray Medical School until 1998.

20. In the last decade this discussion has focused most intensely on the book *The Bell Curve,* which suggests that as a biologically definable group, black children have lower IQs than whites. See Richard J. Herrnstein and Charles Murray, *The Bell Curve: Intelligence and Class Structure in American Life* (New York: Free Press, 1994); Russell Jacoby and Naomi Glauberman, eds., *The*

*Bell Curve Debate: History, Documents, Opinions* (New York: Times Books, 1995).

21. This material, and much of what follows, is easily available in infectious disease textbooks and articles about malaria, such as those listed in note 2 of this chapter. See especially D. J. Weatherall, "Common Genetic Disorders of the Red Cell and the 'Malaria Hypothesis'," *Ann Trop Med Parasitol* 81 (1987): 539–48; F. Fleming, "Abnormal Haemoglobins in the Sudan Savanna of Nigeria," *Ann Trop Med Parasitol* 73 (1979): 161–72; and L. Luca Cavalli-Sforza, Paolo Menozzi, and Alberto Piazza, *The History and Geography of Human Genes* (Princeton, N.J.: Princeton University Press, 1994), 146ff.

22. Martin D. Young et al., "Experimental Testing of the Immunity of Negroes to *Plasmodium vivax,*" *J Parasitol* 41 (1955): 315–18; and Louis H. Miller et al., "Erythrocyte Receptors for (*Plasmodium knowlesi*) Malaria: Duffy Blood Group Determinants," *Science* 189 (1975): 561–63.

23. Corinne Shear Wood, "New Evidence for the Late Introduction of Malaria into the New World," *Curr Anthropol* 16 (1975): 93–104. The phrase "cold screen" is from Marshall T. Newman, "Aboriginal New World Epidemiology and Medical Care, and the Impact of Old World Disease Imports," *Am J Phys Anthropol* 45 (1976): 667–72.

24. Saul Jarcho, "Some Observations on Disease in Prehistoric North America," *Bull Hist Med* 38 (1964): 9; and Bruce-Chwatt, "History of Malaria."

25. David E. Stannard, *American Holocaust: Columbus and the Conquest of the New World* (New York: Oxford University Press, 1992).

26. Alfred W. Crosby, *The Columbian Exchange: Biological and Cultural Consequences of 1492* (Westport, Conn.: Greenwood Press, 1972); and Noble David Cook, *Born to Die: Disease and New World Conquest, 1492–1650* (Cambridge: Cambridge University Press, 1998).

27. Quotations are cited in S. F. Cook, "The Epidemic of 1830–1833 in California and Oregon," *Univ Calif Publ Am Archaeology Ethnol* 43 (1955): 302–26, at 314. See also Robert T. Boyd, "Another Look at the 'Fever and Ague' of Western Oregon," *Ethnohistory* 22 (1975): 135–54; Robert T. Boyd, "Population Decline from Two Epidemics on the Northwest Coast," in John W. Verano and Douglas H. Ubelaker, eds., *Disease and Demography in the Americas* (Washington: Smithsonian Institution Press, 1992); and O. Larsell, *The Doctor in Oregon: A Medical History* (Portland: Oregon Historical Society, 1947).

28. Cited in Herbert J. Forrest, "Malaria and the Union Mission to the Osage Indians, 1820–1837," *Okla State Med J* 69 (1976): 322–27, at 322.

29. Robert Paschal Nespor, "The Ecology of Malaria and Changes in Settlement Pattern on the Cheyenne and Arapaho Reservation, Indian Territory," *Plains Anthropol* 34 (1989): 71–84.

30. On European sources of *vivax* malaria, see Jon Kukla, "Kentish Agues and American Distempers: The Transmission of Malaria from England to Virginia in the Seventeenth Century," *South Stud* 25 (1986): 135–47; J. P. Verhave, "The Advent of Malaria Research in the Netherlands," *Hist Phil Life Sci* 10 (1988): 121–28; Juan Riera Palmero and Anastasio Rojo Vega, "Spanish Agriculture and Malaria in the 18th Century," *Hist Phil Life Sci* 10 (1988): 343–62; Mary J.

Dobson, *Contours of Death and Disease in Early Modern England* (Cambridge: Cambridge University Press, 1997), 287–367; and Leonard Jan Bruce-Chwatt and Julian de Zulueta, *The Rise and Fall of Malaria in Europe: A Historico-epidemiological Study* (Oxford: Oxford University Press, 1980), 131–145. The best analysis of the high mortality when Europeans encountered African parasites is Philip D. Curtin, *Death by Migration: Europe's Encounter with the Tropical World in the Nineteenth Century* (Cambridge: Cambridge University Press, 1989).

31. John Duffy, *Epidemics in Colonial America* (Baton Rouge: Louisiana State University Press, 1953), 202–14.

32. Wyndham B. Blanton, *Medicine in Virginia in the Seventeenth Century* (Richmond: William Byrd Press, 1930), 32–33, 50–55; and Carville V. Earle, "Environment, Disease, and Mortality in Early Virginia," in Thad W. Tate and David L. Ammerman, eds., *The Chesapeake in the Seventeenth Century* (New York: W. W. Norton, 1979), 96–125.

33. Peter Wood, *Black Majority: Negroes in Colonial South Carolina from 1670 through the Stono Rebellion* (New York: Alfred A. Knopf, 1974), 63–91.

34. Peter Coclanis, *The Shadow of a Dream: Economic Life and Death in the South Carolina Low Country, 1670–1920* (New York: Oxford University Press, 1989), 42.

35. H. Roy Merrens and George D. Terry, "Dying in Paradise: Malaria, Mortality, and the Perceptual Environment in Colonial South Carolina," *J South Hist* 50 (1984): 533–50, at 549.

36. Jill Dubisch, "Low Country Fevers: Cultural Adaptations to Malaria in Antebellum South Carolina," *Soc Sci Med* 21 (1985): 641–49; Charles F. Kovacik, "Health Conditions and Town Growth in Colonial and Antebellum South Carolina," *Soc Sci Med.* 12 (1978): 131–36; and St. Julien Ravenel Childs, *Malaria and Colonization in the Carolina Low Country, 1526–1696* (Baltimore: Johns Hopkins University Press, 1940).

37. Darrett B. Rutman and Anita H. Rutman, "Of Agues and Fevers: Malaria in the Early Chesapeake," *Will Mary Q,* 3rd ser., 33 (1976): 31–60.

38. Oliver Wendell Holmes, "Dissertation on Intermittent Fevers in New England," *Boylston Prize Dissertations for the Years 1836 and 1837* (Boston: Charles C. Little and James Brown, 1838).

39. John Duffy, in his *Epidemics in Colonial America,* 202–14, tends to take every reference to ague as evidence of malaria. See also *Oxford English Dictionary,* 2d ed. (Oxford: Clarendon Press, 1989), s.v. "ague."

40. On the early history of cinchona bark, see Saul Jarcho, *Quinine's Predecessor: Francesco Torti and the Early History of Cinchona* (Baltimore and London: Johns Hopkins University Press, 1993).

41. Karen Ordahl Kupperman, "Fear of Hot Climates in the Anglo-American Colonial Experience," *Will Mary Q,* 3rd ser., 41 (1984): 213–40.

42. Philip Curtin, "Epidemiology and the Slave Trade," *Pol Sci Q* 83 (1968): 191–216.

43. John Duffy, "The Impact of Malaria on the South," in Todd L. Savitt and James Harvey Young, eds., *Disease and Distinctiveness in the American South* (Knoxville: University of Tennessee Press, 1988), 29–54, at 36–37.

44. Erwin Ackerknecht, *Malaria in the Upper Mississippi Valley, 1760–1900* (1945; reprint New York: Arno Press, 1977).

CHAPTER TWO: THE MIST RISES

1. Erwin H. Ackerknecht, *Malaria in the Upper Mississippi Valley, 1760–1900* (1945; reprint New York: Arno Press, 1977).

2. David Ramsay, *A Dissertation on the Means of Preserving Health, in Charleston, and the Adjacent Low Country* (Charleston: Markland and M'Iver, 1790), 30.

3. J. C. Nott, "An Examination into the Health and Longevity of the Southern Sea Ports of the United States, with Reference to the Subject of Life Insurance," *South J Med Pharm* 2 (1847): 15.

4. Charles Dickens, *American Notes for General Circulation* (1842; reprint Hammondsworth: Penguin Books, 1972, edited with an introduction by John S. Whitley and Arnold Goldman), 215–16.

5. Charles Dickens, *Martin Chuzzlewit,* edited with an introduction by Margaret Cardwell (Oxford: Clarendon Press, 1982). All page numbers cited in text hereinafter refer to this edition.

6. Frederick Law Olmsted, *The Cotton Kingdom: A Traveler's Observations on Cotton and Slavery in the American Slave States, 1853–1861* (1851; reprint edited with an introduction by Arthur M. Schlesinger, New York: Alfred A. Knopf, 1953).

7. Mark Twain, *Life on the Mississippi* (1883; reprint New York: New American Library, 1961), 316.

8. Andrew McClary, "Don't Go to Michigan, that Land of Ills," *Mich Hist* 67 (1983): 46–48.

9. Charles G. Roland, "'Sunk under the Taxation of Nature': Malaria in Upper Canada," in Charles G. Roland, ed., *Health, Disease and Medicine: Essays in Canadian History* (Toronto: Hannah Institute for the History of Medicine, 1984); and A. Murray Fallis, "Malaria in the 18th and 19th Centuries in Ontario," *Bull Canadian Med Hist* 1 (1984): 25–38.

10. Gert Brieger, "Health and Disease on the Western Frontier: A Bicentennial Appreciation," *West J Med* 125 (1976): 28–35; and Ackerknecht, *Malaria.*

11. Daniel Drake, *Malaria in the Interior Valley of North America*, a selection by Norman D. Levine from *A Systematic Treatise, Historical, Etiological, and Practical, of the Principal Diseases of the Interior Valley of North America . . .* (1850; selection published Urbana: University of Illinois Press, 1964). The page numbers are retained from the original, although large sections have been omitted.

12. Ibid., 703.

13. Ibid., 641.

14.     Ibid., 116.

15.     Dickens, *American Notes*, 224.

16.     Drake, *Malaria*, 324.

17.     Ibid., 323.

18.     Ackerknecht, *Malaria*.

19.     Conevery Bolton, "'The Health of the Country': Body and Environment in the Making of the American West, 1800–1860" (Ph.D. diss., Harvard University, 1998); and Conevery Bolton Valencius, "The Geography of Health and the Making of the American West: Arkansas and Missouri, 1800–1860," in Nicolaas A. Rupke, ed., *Medical Geography in Historical Perspective, Med Hist* Supp. no. 7, forthcoming. Cited with permission of the author.

20.     Drake, *Malaria*, 743–51.

21.     Thomas Findley, "Sappington's Anti-Fever Pills and the Westward Migration," *Trans Clin Climatol Assoc* 79 (1967): 34–44; and W. A. Strickland, "Quinine Pills Manufactured on the Missouri Frontier (1832–1862)," *Pharm Hist* 25 (1983): 61–68.

22.     "Thermaline," patent medicine trade card in the author's possession. My thanks to Ted Kerin for locating this advertisement.

23.     Paul E. Steiner, *Disease in the Civil War* (Springfield, Ill.: Charles C. Thomas, 1968), 10; see also Jeffry S. Sartin, "Infectious Diseases during the Civil War: The Triumph of the 'Third Army,'" *Clin Infect Dis* 16 (1993): 580–84.

24.     Richard A. Gabriel and Karen S. Metz, *A History of Military Medicine*, vol. 2: *From the Renaissance through Modern Times* (New York: Greenwood Press, 1992), 179–96.

25.     Steiner, *Disease*.

26.     Quoted in ibid., 38.

27.     Ibid., 22.

28.     Pascal James Imperato, Howard B. Shookhoff, and Robert P. Harvey, "Malaria in New York City," *N Y St J Med* 73 (1973): 2372–81, 2495–502, 2601–5.

29.     Ackerknecht, *Malaria*.

30.     Ibid., 134–37.

31.     L. W. Hackett, *Malaria in Europe: An Ecological Study* (London: Oxford University Press, 1937), 47–84.

32.     Ackerknecht, *Malaria*, 93–98.

33.     "Ayer's Ague Cure," "Carolina Tolu Tonic," and "Brown's Iron Bitters," advertising cards in the author's possession. My thanks to Ted Kerin, who located these cards for me. The best source of information on the history of patent medicines in the United States remains James Harvey Young, *The Toadstool Millionaires: A Social History of Patent Medicines in America before Federal Regulation* (Princeton, N.J.: Princeton University Press, 1961).

34.     Ackerknecht, *Malaria*, 127.

35.     Ibid., 130.

36.     Charles Rosenberg, *The Cholera Years: The United States in 1832, 1849, and 1866* (Chicago: University of Chicago Press, 1962), 73–75; and John Harley Warner, *The Therapeutic Perspective: Medical Practice, Knowledge, and Identity in America, 1820–1885* (Cambridge, Mass.: Harvard University Press, 1986), 62.

37.     Charles Rosenberg, "The Causes of Cholera: Aspects of Etiological Thought in 19th-century America," *Bull Hist Med* 34 (1960): 331–54.

38.     Joseph Johnston, "Some Accounts of the Origin and Prevention of Yellow Fever in Charleston, S.C.," *Charleston Med J Rev* 4 (1849): 154–69, at 155.

39.     Joel Y. Bell, "Malaria" (M.D. thesis, University of Nashville, 1857), Special Collections, Vanderbilt University Medical Center Library, Nashville, Tenn.; J. K. Mitchell, *On the Cryptogamous Origin of Malarious and Epidemic Fevers* (Philadelphia: Lea and Blanchard, 1849); and Josiah C. Nott, "Yellow Fever Contrasted with Bilious Fever—Reasons for Believing It a Disease Sui Generis—Its Mode of Propagation—Remote Cause—Probably Insect or Animalcular Origin, &c.," *N Orl Med Surg J* 4 (1847–48): 563–601.

40.     J. C. LeHardy, "Yellow Fever. Its History, Causes, Nature, Pathology and Treatment; Considering Exclusively the Epidemic of 1876 in Savannah," *Trans Med Assoc Georgia* 29 (1878): 64–98, at 77.

41.     See, for example, J. W. Compton, "Some Well-Marked Features in the Symptoms and Character of Yellow Fever that Distinguish It from Malarial Fever," *Cinc Lancet Clin* 1 (1878): 185–86.

42.     Margaret Humphreys, *Yellow Fever and the South* (1992; reprint Baltimore: Johns Hopkins University Press, 1998).

43.     J. C. Faget, "A Reply to an Article by Dr. Delery," *N Orl J Med* 23 (1870): 759–77, at 767. See also J. C. Faget, "Haematemesic Paludal Fever, Observed at New Orleans," *N Orl J Med* 23 (1870): 440–59.

44.     James Harris, "An Essay on the Climate and Fevers of the Southwestern, Southern, Atlantic, and Gulf States, " *N Orl J Med* 23 (1870): 401–40; R. Charles Delery, "Brief Remarks upon Dr. Faget's Malarial Catarral Hemorrhagic Fever," *N Orl J Med* 23 (1870): 222–23; "Letter from Sam'l H. Coffman of Enterprise, Miss.," *N Orl J Med* 23 (1870): 795–97.

45.     Dale C. Smith, "The Rise and Fall of Typhomalarial Fever," *J Hist Med Allied Sci* 37 (1982): 182–220, 287–321.

46.     Margaret Warner (Humphreys), "Hunting the Yellow Fever Germ: The Principle and Practice of Etiological Proof in Late Nineteenth-century America," *Bull Hist Med* 59 (1985): 361–82.

47.     Gordon Harrison, *Mosquitoes, Malaria and Man: A History of the Hostilities since 1880* (New York: E. P. Dutton, 1978), 7–16.

48.     Dale C. Smith and Lorraine B. Sanford, "Laveran's Germ: The Reception and Use of a Medical Discovery," *Am J Trop Med Hyg* 34 (1985): 2–20.

49.     Joseph Parrish, "Address by the President: The Geography of Malaria," *Trans Med Soc N J* (1886), 39–52, at 39. For a detailed discussion of the words *malaria* and *malarial* just as they were changing meaning, see George M. Sternberg, *Malaria and Malarial Diseases* (New York: William Wood & Co., 1884).

50. Harrison, *Mosquitoes, Malaria, and Man,* 102–8; personal communication, Bernardino Fantini and William Bynum, April 1996. A recent biography of Ross is Edwin R. Nye and Mary E. Gibson, *Ronald Ross, Malariologist and Polymath: A Biography* (New York: St. Martin's Press, 1997). For the Italian point of view, see Ernesto Capanna, ed., "Battista Grassi, uno Zoologo per la Malaria," *Parassitologia,* 38, supp. 1 (1996): 1–47.

51. Robert Koch, "Erster Bericht über die Thätigkeit der Malariaexpedition," *Deutsche Med Woch* 25 (1899), 601–4; Robert Koch, "Zweiter Bericht über die Thätigkeit der Malariaexpedition," *Deutsche Med Woch* 26 (1900): 88–90; Robert Koch, "Dritter Bericht über die Thätigkeit der Malariaexpedition," *Deutsche Med Woch* 26 (1900): 281–84; Robert Koch, "Fünfter Bericht über die Thätigkeit der Malariaexpedition," *Deutsche Med Woch* 26 (1900): 541–42; Robert Koch, "Zusammenfassende Darstellung der Ergebnisse der Malariaexpedition," *Deutsche Med Woch* 26 (1900): 781–83.

52. On Koch's impact, see, for example, Theobald Smith, "The Sources Favoring Conditions and Prophylaxis of Malaria in Temperate Climates with Special Reference to Massachusetts," *Bos Med Surg J* 149 (1903): 57–64, 87–92, 115–18, 139–44, at 61–62; and William Kraus, "What We Should Know about Malaria Disease," *South Med J* 1 (1908): 25–32, 90–95, 141–46, at 27.

53. William H. Deaderick and Loyd Thompson, *The Endemic Diseases of the Southern States* (Philadelphia: W. B. Saunders, 1916), 36. For a similar reliance on Koch concerning carriers and childhood infections, see R. H. von Ezdorf, "Endemic Index of Malaria in the United States," *Public Health Rep* 31 (1916): 819–28, at 819.

54. L. O. Howard, *Mosquitoes; How They Live; How They Carry Disease; How They Are Classified; How They May Be Destroyed* (New York: McClure, Phillips & Co., 1901).

55. Harrison, *Mosquitoes, Malaria and Man,* 157–68.

CHAPTER THREE: RACE, POVERTY, AND PLACE

1. Gordon Harrison, *Mosquitoes, Malaria and Man: A History of the Hostilities since 1880* (New York: E. P. Dutton, 1978), 171–76.

2. W. V. King and G. H. Bradley, "Distribution of the Nearctic Species of Anopheles," in Forest Ray Moulton, ed., *A Symposium on Human Malaria with Special Reference to North America and the Caribbean Region* (Washington, D.C.: American Association for the Advancement of Science, 1941), 71–78; S. T. Darling, "Discussion on Relative Importance in Transmitting Malaria of Anopheles quadrimaculatus, punctipennis, and crucians and Advisability of Differentiating Between These Species in Applying Control Measures," *South Med J* 18 (1925): 452–58.

3. L.W. Hackett, *Malaria in Europe: An Ecological Study* (London: Oxford University Press, 1937), 61–64.

4. F. W. O'Connor, "Biologic Investigations," *South Med J* 17 (1924): 599–602; S.T. Darling, "Discussion on the Relative Importance"; S.T. Darling, "Entomological Research in Malaria," *South Med J* 18 (1925): 446–49; Paul S. Carley and Marshall Balfour, "Prevalence of Malaria in Humphreys and Sunflower

Counties, Mississippi, in 1927–28," *South Med J* 22 (1929): 377–82; Tennessee Valley Authority, *Malaria and Its Control in the Tennessee Valley* (Chattanooga: Tennessee Valley Authority, 1941), 11.

5.  G. H. Bradley and W. V. King, "Bionomics and Ecology of Nearctic Anopheles," in Moulton, ed., *Symposium on Human Malaria,* 79–87.

6.  James Stevens Simmons, "The Transmission of Malaria by the Anopheles Mosquitoes of North America," in Moulton, ed., *Symposium on Human Malaria,* 113–30.

7.  Hackett, *Malaria in Europe,* 68.

8.  L. D. Fricks, "Malaria Control in the U.S.: Retrospect and Prospect," *South Med J* 17 (1924): 578–82, at 580.

9.  Mark F. Boyd, "An Historical Sketch of the Prevalence of Malaria in North America," *Am J Trop Med Hyg* 21 (1941): 223–44, 237.

10. Kenneth F. Maxcy, "Spleen Rate of School Boys in the Mississippi Delta," *Public Health Rep* 38 (1923): 2466–72, at 2467.

11. C. L. Van Dine, "The Losses of Rural Industries through Mosquitoes that Convey Malaria," *South Med J* 8 (1915): 184–94.

12. Mark F. Boyd and Gerald Ponton, "The Recent Distribution of Malaria in the Southeastern United States," *Am J Trop Med* 13 (1933): 143–66; and Robert B. Watson and E. L. Spain, Jr., "Studies on Malaria in the Tennessee Valley: The Influence of Physiography on the Occurrence of Breeding Places of Anopheles quadrimaculatus in Northern Alabama," *Am J Trop Med* 17 (1937): 289–305.

13. Kenneth F. Maxcy, "Epidemiological Principles Affecting the Distribution of Malaria in the Southern U.S.," *Public Health Rep* 39 (1924) 1113–27, at 1117.

14. "The Southern Farmer's Burden," cartoon, in Photographic Collection, Records of the USPHS, Record Group 90, NACP.

15. M. A. Barber et al., "Malaria in the Prairie Rice Regions of Louisiana and Arkansas," *Public Health Rep* 41 (1926) 2527–49, at 2544, 2547.

16. Marshall A. Barber, *A Malariologist in Many Lands* (Lawrence: University of Kansas Press, 1946), 16.

17. The "butter on bread" analogy comes from L. L. Williams, quoted in "School Pupils Shock Troops in Battle Against Malaria," *Sci News Let,* Nov. 6, 1937, 294–95.

18. Sheila Zurbrigg, "Did Starvation Protect from Malaria? Distinguishing between Severity and Lethality of Infectious Disease in Colonial India," *Soc Sci Hist* 21 (1997): 27–58. Mary J. Dobson also discusses this controversy in her *Contours of Death and Disease in Early Modern England* (Cambridge: Cambridge University Press, 1997), 287–367.

19. J. B. Ascanio-Rodriguez, "Malaria and Hookworm in Venezuela," *South Med J* 23 (1930): 426; and Henry Hansen, "Hookworm and Malaria," *South Med J* 23 (1930): 426–28.

20. "Screens and Health," *Health Bull (NC)* 30, 4 (1915), 84–85. On screening as a part of cleanliness, see Nancy Tomes, *The Gospel of Germs: Men, Women, and*

the *Microbe in American Life* (Cambridge, Mass.: Harvard University Press, 1998), and Naomi Rogers, *Dirt and Disease: Polio before FDR* (New Brunswick, N.J.: Rutgers University Press, 1992).

21. Harry Beckman, "The Prophylaxis of Malaria," *South Med J* 33 (1940): 516–22, at 517.

22. Paul F. Russell, *Man's Mastery of Malaria* (London: Oxford University Press, 1955), 154–157, at 179.

23. Martin D. Young et al., "The Infectivity of Native Malarias in South Carolina to *Anopheles quadrimaculatus*," *Am J Trop Med* 28 (1948): 303–11, at 309.

24. Frederick L. Hoffman, "Race Traits and Tendencies of the American Negro," *Publications American Economic Association* 11 (1896), 1–139, at v.

25. Ibid., 314, 231.

26. The literature on the history of the eugenics movement is rich and abundant. See, for example, Daniel J. Kevles, *In the Name of Eugenics: Genetics and the Uses of Human Heredity,* rev. ed. (Cambridge, Mass.: Harvard University Press, 1995); Stephen Jay Gould, *The Mismeasure of Man,* rev. ed. (New York: W. W. Norton, 1996); and Edward J. Larson, *Sex, Race, and Science: Eugenics in the Deep South* (Baltimore: Johns Hopkins Press, 1995).

27. Hoffman, "Race Traits," 63, 95.

28. See, for example, J. C. Nott, *The Negro Race. Its Ethnology and History* (Mobile. Ala.: Mobile Daily Press, 1866), 25; and William Benjamin Smith, *The Color Line: A Brief in Behalf of the Unborn* (New York: McClure, Phillips & Co., 1905), 58, 192, 217, 228. On the infamous Jarvis census, see Gerald N. Grob, *Edward Jarvis and the Medical World of Nineteenth Century America* (Knoxville: University of Tennessee Press, 1978), 71–75.

29. Marvin L. Graves, "The Negro a Menace to the Health of the White Race," *South Med J* 9 (1916): 407–13.

30. C. Jeff Miller, "Special Medical Problems of the Colored Woman," *South Med J* 25 (1932): 733–39, at 733–34.

31. L. C. Allen, "The Negro Health Problem," *Am J Public Health* 5 (1915): 194–203, at 194, 196.

32. *Conference for the Betterment of Health Conditions among Negroes, called by the Louisana State Board of Health New Orleans, April 24, 1914* (New Orleans: Louisiana State Board of Health, 1914), 3.

33. On Typhoid Mary, see Judith Walzer Leavitt, *Typhoid Mary: Captive to the Public's Health* (Boston: Beacon Press, 1996). David S. Barnes, *The Making of a Social Disease: Tuberculosis in Nineteenth-Century France* (Berkeley: University of California Press, 1995), is one of several recent and excellent books on tuberculosis and contains a particularly memorable account of the war on spitting. For the general history of the concept of carriers, Charles-Edward-Amory Winslow, *The Conquest of Epidemic Disease: A Chapter in the History of Ideas* (1943; reprint Madison: University of Wisconsin Press, 1980), 337–46, has not yet been surpassed. Classic articles on the discovery of the carrier have been reprinted in *The Carrier State* (New York: Arno Press, 1977).

34. Robert Koch, "Erster Bericht über die Thätigkeit der Malariaexpedition," *Deutsche Med Woch* 25 (1899), 601–604; Robert Koch, "Zweiter Bericht über die Thätigkeit der Malariaexpedition," *Deutsche Med Woch* 26 (1900): 88–90; Robert Koch, "Dritter Bericht über die Thätigkeit der Malariaexpedition," *Deutsche Med Woch* 26 (1900): 281–84; Robert Koch, "Fünfter Bericht über die Thätigkeit der Malariaexpedition," *Deutsche Med Woch* 26 (1900): 541–42; Robert Koch, "Zusammenfassende Darstellung der Ergebnisse der Malariaexpedition," *Deutsche Med Woch* 26 (1900): 781–83.

35. See, for example, the popular malaria textbook, William H. Deaderick, *A Practical Study of Malaria* (Philadelphia: W. H. Saunders, 1909), 50–54.

36. C. C. Bass, "A Discussion of Malaria Carriers and the Important Role They Play in the Persistence and Spread of Malaria," *South Med J* 8 (1915): 182–84.

37. Maxcy, "Spleen Rate."

38. Adapted from M. A. Barber et al., "Prevalence of Malaria (1925) in Parts of Delta of Mississippi and Arkansas: Economic Conditions," *South Med J* 19 (1926): 373–77; M. A. Barber and Bruce Mayne, "The Seasonal Incidence of Malaria Parasites in the Southern United States," *South Med J* 17 (1924): 583–91; R. H. von Ezdorf, "Endemic Index of Malaria in the United States," *Public Health Rep* 31 (1916): 819–28; H. A. Taylor, "The Investigation and Control of Malaria in Pamlico County, North Carolina," *Health Bull (NC)* 38 (Aug. 1923): 5–10; T.H.D. Griffitts, "Malaria Control by Use of Paris Green: Preliminary Report on County-wide Work in Dougherty Co., Georgia," *South Med J* 23 (1930): 428–34.

39. Mary Gover, "Negro Mortality," *Public Health Rep* 61 (1946): 259–65, 1529–38; 63 (1948): 201–13; and 66 (1951): 295–305.

40. Julian Herman Lewis, *The Biology of the Negro* (Chicago: University of Chicago Press, 1942), 192–95.

41. Hoffman, "Race Traits," 105.

42. A. G. Fort, "The Negro Health Problem in Rural Communities," *Am J Public Health* 5 (1915): 191–93; W. E. Burghardt DuBois, *The Health and Physique of the Negro American* (Atlanta: University of Atlanta Press, 1906); James A. Doull, "Comparative Racial Immunity to Diseases," *J Negro Educ* 6 (1937): 429–37; and H. A. Poindexter, "Special Health Problems of Negroes in Rural Areas," *J Negro Educ* 6 (1937): 399–412.

43. Kenneth Maxcy, Wilson G. Smilie, and W. A. Plecker, "Malaria Statistics," *South Med J* 18 (1925): 449–52.

44. On the history of syphilis, see Allan M. Brandt, *No Magic Bullet: A Social History of Venereal Disease in the United States since 1880* (New York and Oxford: Oxford University Press, 1985); and Claude Quétel, *History of Syphilis,* trans. Judith Braddock and Brian Pike (Baltimore: Johns Hopkins University Press, 1990).

45. Joel Braslow, *Mental Ills and Bodily Cures: Psychiatric Treatment in the First Half of the Twentieth Century* (Berkeley: University of California Press, 1997), 71–94.

46. Bruce Mayne, "Some Recent Investigations of the Viability and Longevity of the Malaria Parasite in the Mosquito as Related to Malaria Therapy of Paresis," *South Med J* 25 (1932): 549–51.

47. Mark Boyd, Diary for the Second Quarter, 1931, entries for May and June, Folder 468, Box 48, Record Group 1, Series 100, Rockefeller Foundation Archives, RAC; Mark Boyd and Warren K. Stratman-Thomas, "Studies on Benign Tertian Malaria: 4. On the Refractoriness of Negroes to Inoculation with Plasmodium vivax," *Am J Hyg* 18 (1933): 485–89; Frederic Becker, Lawrence I. Kaplan, Hilton S. Read, and Mark F. Boyd, "Variations in Susceptibility to Therapeutic Malaria," *Am J Med Sci* 211 (1946): 680–85.

48. A. C. Allison, "Protection Afforded by Sickle-Cell Trait against Subtertian Malarial Infection," *Br Med J* 1 (1954): 290–94; A. C. Allison, "The Distribution of the Sickle-Cell Trait in East Africa and Elsewhere, and Its Apparent Relationship to the Incidence of Subtertian Malaria," *Trans R Soc Trop Med Hyg* 48 (1954): 312–18; and F. Fleming, "Abnormal Haemoglobins in the Sudan Savanna of Nigeria," *Ann Trop Med Parasitol* 73 (1979): 161–72. On the history of sickle-cell anemia, see Keith Wailoo, *Drawing Blood: Technology and Disease Identity in Twentieth-Century America* (Baltimore: Johns Hopkins University Press, 1997), 134–61; and Melbourne Tapper, "An 'Anthropathology' of the 'American Negro': Anthropology, Genetics, and the New Racial Science, 1940–1952," *Soc Hist Med* 10 (1997): 263–89.

49. Barber, *A Malariologist in Many Lands*, 9.

CHAPTER FOUR: MAKING MALARIA CONTROL PROFITABLE

1. On this period, see, for example, Barbara Gutmann Rosenkrantz, *Public Health and the State: Changing Views in Massachusetts, 1842–1936* (Cambridge, Mass.: Harvard University Press, 1972); Allan Brandt, *No Magic Bullet: A Social History of Venereal Disease in the United States since 1880* (New York: Oxford University Press, 1985); René and Jean Dubos, *The White Plague: Tuberculosis, Man, and Society* (1952; reprint New Brunswick, N.J.: Rutgers University Press, 1987); Margaret Humphreys, *Yellow Fever and the South* (1992; reprint Johns Hopkins University Press, 1998); and James Harvey Young, *Pure Food: Securing the Federal Food and Drug Act of 1906* (Princeton, N.J.: Princeton University Press, 1989).

2. Joseph Kesserling, *Arsenic and Old Lace* (New York: Random House, 1941). In the play the delusional character Teddy believes he is digging the Panama Canal in the basement and worries about the yellow fever down there.

3. Gordon Harrison, *Mosquitoes, Malaria and Man: A History of the Hostilities since 1880* (New York: E. P. Dutton, 1978), 157–68.

4. There are many valuable sources on southern history during this era. Perhaps most useful are William A. Link, *The Paradox of Southern Progressivism, 1880–1930* (Chapel Hill: University of North Carolina Press, 1992); James C. Cobb, *The Most Southern Place on Earth: The Mississippi Delta and the Roots of Regional Identity* (Oxford: Oxford University Press, 1992); and George B. Tindall, *The Emergence of the New South: 1913–1945* (Baton Rouge: Louisiana State University Press, 1967).

5.      Franklin D. Roosevelt to the Members of the Conference on Economic Condi-
        tions in the South, July 5, 1938; reprinted in National Emergency Council,
        *Report on Economic Conditions of the South* (n.p., 1938), 1–2, at 1.

6.      This tie between malaria and poor agricultural production was made explicit
        in a 1943 educational film about malaria. It showed, in cartoon format, a cheer-
        ful farm shriveling to a dark ruin once the previously prosperous farmer is
        struck with malaria. *The Mosquito,* National Archives and Record Service 18 C
        157, Official Training film, Medical Department, U.S. Army. The film was
        originally produced by Walt Disney Studios in collaboration with the coordi-
        nator of inter-American affairs. The version in my possession is clearly a war
        training film. Another version entitled *The Winged Scourge* is in the Nelson
        Rockefeller papers of RAC. Rockefeller was the coordinator of inter-American
        affairs during World War II, and this film was distributed in Latin America as a
        goodwill gesture on the part of the U.S. government.

7.      Humphreys, *Yellow Fever and the South.*

8.      John Ettling, *The Germ of Laziness: Rockefeller Philanthropy and Public
        Health in the New South* (Cambridge, Mass.: Harvard University Press, 1981).

9.      Elizabeth W. Etheridge, *The Butterfly Caste: A Social History of Pellagra in the
        South* (Westport, Conn.: Greenwood, 1972).

10.     Philip D. Curtin, "Medical Knowledge and Urban Planning in Tropical
        Africa," *Am Hist Rev* 90 (1985): 594–613.

11.     John W. Cell, "Anglo-Indian Medical Theory and the Origins of Segregation
        in West Africa," *Am Hist Rev* 91 (1986): 307–35.

12.     John W. Cell, *The Highest Stage of White Supremacy: The Origins of Segrega-
        tion in South Africa and the American South* (Cambridge: Cambridge Univer-
        sity Press, 1982).

13.     Harrison, *Mosquitoes, Malaria and Man,* 170–72.

14.     R. H. von Ezdorf, "Demonstrations of Malaria Control," *Public Health Rep*
        31(1916): 614–27, at 624.

15.     "Results Obtained by a Local Community following Anti-mosquito Demon-
        stration Studies by the United States Public Health Service in Cooperation
        with the International Health Board," *Public Health Rep* 33 (1918): 1154–58.

16.     Charles Cassedy Bass Papers, Manuscript Collections, Howard-Tilton Memo-
        rial Library, Tulane University, New Orleans, La.

17.     "Treatment of Malaria," *Public Health Rep* 34 (1919): 2959–60.

18.     C. C. Bass, "Studies on Malaria Control. III. Observations of the Prevalence of
        Malaria, and Its Control by Treating Malaria Carriers in a Locality of Great
        Prevalence in the Mississippi Delta," *South Med J* 12 (1919): 190–93.

19.     Interview with Dr. C. C. Bass, New Orleans, November 1950, notes by Lewis
        W. Hackett for IHB History, Record Group 3.1, Series 908, Box 3, vol. 1,
        pp. 281–82, at 282, RAC.

20.     C. C. Bass, comments following L. D. Fricks, "The Malaria Awakening of the
        South," *J Am Med Assoc* 75 (1920): 847–51, at 850.

21. *Health Bull Mississippi St Bd Health* 9 (April 1921); L. D. Fricks to Surgeon General, Apr. 12, 1922, in Folder for April 1922, Box 477, Central File 1897–1923, Records of the USPHS, Record Group 90, NACP.

22. T.H.D. Griffitts, "Eight Weeks' Quinine Treatment for Malaria," *Public Health Rep* 40 (1925): 539–48.

23. By the time Hackett interviewed him in 1950, Bass could say of his "standard therapy" that in design it was good, but that the drug quinine was just not powerful enough to make it work. But he stopped publishing on the subject after the 1920s, so it is difficult to determine at what point he actually admitted failure.

24. Griffitts, "Eight Weeks' Quinine," 539–48.

25. Comments of Roy K. Flanagan, following R. K. Collins, "An Experience with Intensive Quinine Treatment under Field Conditions," *South Med J* 19 (1926): 383–92.

26. Mark Boyd, "Studies of the Epidemiology of Malaria in the Coastal Lowlands of Brazil, Made before and after the Execution of Control Measures," *Am J Hyg* Monograph Series no. 5, 1926.

27. H. R. Carter, "Resume of Methods for Control of Malaria: Indications; Results; Costs," *Am J Public Health* 10 (1920): 528–32, at 531–32.

28. Ennion G. Williams, "Rural Malaria Control with the County as the Unit," *South Med J* 15 (1922): 362–68, at 363.

29. T.H.D. Griffitts, comments following ibid., 366.

30. W. E. Deeks, comments following T.H.D. Griffitts, "Malaria Control by Use of Paris Green: Preliminary Report on County-wide Work in Dougherty Co., Ga.," *South Med J* 23 (1930): 428–34, at 433–34. See also W. E. Deeks, "Recent Developments in the Control of Malaria," *South Med J* 23 (1930): 417–20.

31. M. A. Fort, comments following Griffitts, "Malaria Control by Use of Paris Green," 434.

32. L. W. Hackett, *Malaria in Europe: An Ecological Study* (1937; reprint London: Oxford University Press, 1944), 177–97, 288.

33. W. V. King, "Historical Developments and Progress in Our Knowledge of Malaria Control," *South Med J* 31 (1938): 797–802, at 801.

34. Herbert C. Clark and William H. W. Komp, "A Summary of Ten Years of Observations on Malaria in Panama with Reference to Control with Quinine, Atabrine, and Plasmochin, without Anti-mosquito Measures," in Forest Ray Moulton, ed., *A Symposium on Human Malaria with Special Reference to North America and the Caribbean Region* (Washington: American Association for the Advancement of Science, 1941), 273–84; H. C. Clark, W.H.W. Komp, and D. M. Jobbins, "A Tenth Year's Observations on Malaria in Panama, with Reference to the Occurrence of Variations in the Parasite Index, during Continued Treatment with Atabrine and Plasmochine," *Am J Trop Med* 21 (1941): 191–216.

35. Wickliffe Rose, "Malaria Control," *J Am Med Assoc* 73 (1919): 1414–20; Charles W. Garrison, comments following R. C. Derivaux, "Some Results of Malaria

Control by Control of the Insect Host: Public Health and Economic Aspects," *South Med J* 11 (1918): 556–62, at 561–62.

36. L. D. Fricks, "Malaria Control in the U. S.: Retrospect and Prospect," *South Med J* 17 (1924): 578–82.

37. J. L. Bowman, comments following J. A. LePrince, "Feasibility of Advocating Building Designs or Regulations in Reference to Mosquito Control," *South Med J* 18 (1925): 465–66, at 466.

38. T.H.D. Griffitts, comments following Williams, "Rural Malaria Control," 466.

39. D. L. Van Dine, "Mosquito Work of the Bureau of Entomology," *Am J Public Health* 10 (1920): 116–19, at 119.

40. L. L. Williams, "Rural Malaria Control," *Health Bull (NC)* 39 (1924): 24–27, at 26.

41. Walter Rowland, narrative, FWP-SHC.

42. The Commission for the Study and Prevention of Malaria to John D. Rockefeller, Oct. 1, 1913, Proposal for Rockefeller Foundation to Fund Malaria campaign, Central File 1897–1923, Malaria, 1913, Records of the USPHS, Record Group 90, NACP. On the broader application of this argument in other countries and its use as a cultural construct, see Peter J. Brown, "Malaria, *Miseria,* and Underpopulation in Sardinia: The 'Malaria Blocks Development' Cultural Model," *Med Anthropol* 17 (1997): 239–54.

43. R. H. von Ezdorf, "Demonstrations of Malaria Control," *Public Health Rep* 31 (1916): 614–27, at 621, 624.

44. H. H. Smiley, "What the Cotton Belt Railway Company Is Doing for the Prevention of Malaria," *South Med J* 11 (1913): 576–77; W. H. Van Hovenberg, "The Bearing of Malaria on Railroad Operation," *South Med J* 11 (1918): 562–69; S. W. Beach, Illinois Central Railroad, comments following S. W. Welch, "Development of Malaria Control Work in Alabama on a County-wide Basis," *South Med J* 16 (1923): 260–68, 268.

45. W. H. Van Hovenberg, "The Control of Malaria for a Railroad System, Based on the Experience of the St. Louis Southwestern during 1917, 1918, 1919," *South Med J* 13 (1920): 418–23, at 418.

46. Van Hovenberg, "Bearing of Malaria."

47. Henry W. Stanley, "Public Health as a Business Proposition," *South Med J* 25 (1932): 665–71.

48. E. B. Johnson, comments following S. W. Welch, "Direct and Indirect Advantages of Urban Malaria Control to State Health Program," *South Med J* 15 (1922): 358–61, at 361.

49. Frank R. Shaw, comments following Welch, "Direct and Indirect," 361.

50. J. L. Bowman, comments following J. A. LePrince, "Feasibility of Advocating Building Designs or Regulations in Reference to Mosquito Control," *South Med J* 18 (1925): 465–66, at 466.

51. H. A. Johnson, "The Importance of Plantation Malaria to Memphis and the Plantation Owner," *South Med J* 21 (1928): 780.

52. Howard R. Fullerton, "Screening and Mosquito Proofing as Elements in Malaria Control," *Am J Public Health* 21 (1931): 382–87, at 383.

53. F. J. Underwood, comments following M. A. Barber, W.H.W. Komp, and T. B. Hayne, "Prevalence of Malaria (1925) in Parts of the Delta of Mississippi and Arkansas: Economic Conditions," *South Med J* 19 (1926): 373–77, at 376–77.

54. D. L. Van Dine, "The Losses to Rural Industries through Mosquitoes that Convey Malaria," *South Med J* 8 (1915): 184–94; D. L. Van Dine, "Mosquito Work of the Bureau of Entomology," *Am J Public Health* 10 (1920): 116–19.

55. Walter H. Voskuil, *The Economics of Water Power Development* (New York: McGraw-Hill, 1928), 90–91; George B. Tindall, *The Emergence of the New South 1913–1945* (Baton Rouge: Louisiana State University Press, 1967), 72.

56. T.H.D. Griffitts, "Impounded Waters and Malaria," *South Med J* 19 (1926): 367–70, 368.

57. H. R. Carter, "The Effect of Variation of Level of Impounded Water on the Control of Anopheles Production," *South Med J* 17 (1924): 575–78, at 575.

58. Griffitts, "Impounded Waters," 368.

59. Voskuil, *Economics of Water Power*, 138, 171–73.

60. Ibid., 157.

61. S. W. Welch, comments following Carter, "Effect of Variation," 577.

62. Carter, "Effect of Variation," 575–76.

63. H. R. Carter, "The Effect of Impounded Water on the Incidence of Malaria," *South Med J* 8 (1915): 173–82; Carter, "Effect of Variation"; and E. H. Gage, "Studies of Impounded Waters in Relation to Malaria," *Public Health Rep* 40 (1925): 1357–75.

64. See the correspondence of F. D. Fricks, H. R. Carter, J. A. LePrince, and S. W. Welch in the Folders for 1919–23, Boxes 475–79, Central Files 1899–1923, Records of the USPHS, Record Group 90, NACP.

65. S. W. Welch, comments following W. G. Smillie, "Further Studies of the Impounded Area at Gantt, Alabama," *South Med J* 20 (1927): 475–80, at 478. See also S. W. Welch, "Development of Malaria Control Work in Alabama on a County-wide Basis," *South Med J* 16 (1923): 260–68; S. W. Welch, "Malaria Control Activities in Alabama," *South Med J* 19 (1926): 397–99; W. G. Smillie, "Studies of an Epidemic of Malaria at the Gantt Impounded Area, Covington County, Alabama," *Am J Hyg* 7 (1927): 40–72.

66. M. A. Fort, comments following Smillie, "Further Studies," 479.

67. A. T. McCormack, comments following L. T. Coggleshall, "Report of a Malaria Survey and Control Methods on Lake Murray, Columbia, S.C.," *South Med J* 23 (1930): 442–45, at 445.

68. T. F. Abercrombie, "Malaria Control in Georgia for the Year 1928," *South Med J* 22 (1929): 405.

69. F. M. Boldridge, comments following D. Clark, "Methods and Approximate Costs of Malarial Preventive Measures on High Rock Lake in North Carolina," *South Med J* 24 (1931): 442–49, at 446.

70. Boldridge, comments following Clark, "Methods," 447.

71. W. G. Stromquist, comments following Smillie, "Further Studies," 477.

72. Bob and Christine Curtis, narrative, FWP-SHC. This story is drawn from a Federal Writers' Project interview. The speech appears as the interviewer recorded it. Although the use of dialect may seem old-fashioned or even offensive to some, this is how it appears in the original, and I chose not to change it. For a discussion of the Federal Writers' Project and the potential biases and weaknesses of its narratives, see Chapter 6.

CHAPTER FIVE: "A DITCH IN TIME SAVES QUININE?"

1. Thomas J. Leblanc, "Malaria," *American Mercury* (Sept. 1924): 366–71, quoted in "Malaria in Southern Georgia," *Am J Public Health* 14 (1924): 1037.

2. L. M. Clarkson, "Malaria Control in Georgia," *South Med J* 23 (1930): 462–63, at 463.

3. Frederick L. Hoffman, "Malaria in Mississippi and Adjacent States," *South Med J* 25 (1932): 657–62, at 662. Hoffman was one of the founders of the National Malaria Committee, a group of physicians, entomologists, sanitary engineers, and statisticians who gathered to discuss malaria during the annual meeting of the Southern Medical Association. He is also remembered for claiming that the black race would ultimately become extinct because of innate weaknesses in its stock. His skills as a prognosticator thus failed more than once.

4. Louis L. Williams, "The Anti-malaria Program in North America," in Forest Ray Moulton, ed., *A Symposium on Human Malaria with Special Reference to North America and the Caribbean Region* (Washington, D.C.: American Association for the Advancement of Science, 1941), 365–70.

5. Ernest Carroll Faust, "Clinical and Public Health Aspects of Malaria in the United States from an Historical Perspective," *Am J Trop Med* 25 (1945): 185–201, at 191.

6. See Chapter 6.

7. Kenneth Maxcy, "Malaria Statistics," *South Med J* 18 (1925): 449–52; Justin Andrews, "General Considerations in Planning Malaria Control," in Moulton, ed., *Symposium on Human Malaria,* 285–94; Robert Briggs Watson and Margaret E. Rice, "Notes on the Morbidity of Naturally Occurring Malaria," *J Nat Malaria Soc* 57 (1946): 7–12, at 12.

8. Frederick L. Hoffman, "Modern Aspects of Malaria Problems in Peace and War," *South Med J* 11 (1918): 545–51, at 545.

9. K. B. Humphreys, Jr., personal communication, August 1994.

10. Alban Papineau, "Chronic Malaria," *N C Med J* 7 (1946): 153–60, at 154. The MCWA report for 1943–44 noted another instance in which all the reported cases from 1939 to 1943 were white, and malaria deaths from the same period were black (p. 9). This was cited not as a biological racial phenomenon but as a measure of differences in reporting regarding racial groups, without further analysis as to its basis.

11.  "Malaria Incidence 1934–5," *South Med J* 28 (1935): 765; Henry Hanson et al., "Some Factors in the Epidemiology of Malaria," *Am J Public Health* 25 (1935): 156–61; and Louis L. Williams, Jr., "Civil Works Administration Emergency Relief Administration Malaria Control Programs in the South," *Am J Public Health* 25 (1935): 11–14.

12.  Robert Briggs Watson et al., "A Review of Malaria Studies and Control in the Tennessee Valley in 1945," *J Nat Malaria Soc* 5 (1946): 193–203, at 193; and Williams, "Civil Works," 14.

13.  C. M. White and L. L. Parks, "Malaria Studies and Investigations in North Carolina," *N C Med J* 1(1940): 92–94; and H. F. Schoof and D. F. Ashton, "The Decline and Last Recorded Outbreaks of Malaria in North Carolina," *J Nat Malaria Soc* 10 (1951): 306–16.

14.  *Malaria Control in War Areas, 1942–43* (Washington: U.S. Public Health Service, 1943), 10; Alban Papineau, "Chronic Malaria," *N C Med J* 7 (1946): 153–60, at 157; and Justin M. Andrews et al., "Malaria Eradication in the United States," *Am J Public Health* 40 (1950): 1405–11, at 1409.

15.  *Malaria Control in War Areas 1945–46* (Washington: U.S. Public Health Service, 1946), 63; and George H. Bradley and Melvin H. Goodwin, Jr., "Malaria Observation Stations of the Public Health Service," *J Nat Malaria Soc* 8 (1949): 181–91. The *CDC Bulletins* from 1947 to 1951 frequently comment on the Newton, Georgia, station's anopheles mosquito research and the lack of malaria cases in spite of repeated blood smear surveys in the nearby communities.

16.  Thomas Kirkwood, "The Recrudescence of Malaria," *Ill Med J* 71 (1937): 58–63, at 61.

17.  See, for example, W. Scott Johnson, "Malaria Control in Missouri in 1932," *South Med J* 26 (1933): 472; J. N. Baker, "Malaria Control in Alabama in 1932," *South Med J* 26 (1933): 469; E. L. Bishop, "Malaria Control in Tennessee," *South Med J* 27 (1934): 656–57; J. N. Baker, "Malaria Control in Alabama," *South Med J* 27 (1934): 651–52; and J. A. O'Hara, "Malaria Control in Louisiana in 1933," *South Med J* 27 (1934): 654–55.

18.  L. M. Clarkson, "Malaria Control in Georgia by Convict Labor," *South Med J* 26 (1933): 461–65, at 461.

19.  Louis L. Williams, "Civil Works Administration, Emergency Relief Administration Malaria Control Program in the South," *Am J Public Health* 25 (1935): 11–14.

20.  Frank Sullivan included "the shovel brigade" among standard catchphrases about the WPA in "The Cliche Expert Testifies as a Roosevelt Hater" (1938), reprinted in William E. Leuchtenburg, *The New Deal: A Documentary History* (Columbia: University of South Carolina Press, 1968), 208. On the New Deal in general, Leuchtenburg's *Franklin Roosevelt and the New Deal* (New York: Harper and Row, 1963) remains the standard reference.

21.  "WPA Workers Fight Mosquitoes," *Am City* (Oct. 1936): 51–52.

22.  L. L. Williams, "Report of the Subcommittee on Malaria Prevention Activities, 1937," *South Med J* 31 (1938): 818–19.

23. E. L. Bishop, "The Part Played by a County Health Department in the Ultimate Control of Rural Malaria," *South Med J* 26 (1933): 447–48.

24. "Malaria," *South Med J* 26 (1933): 474.

25. W. N. Bispham, "Malaria in the Southern States," *South Med J* 32 (1939): 848–51, at 850.

26. This speed and lack of surveys was reported from state after state. See, for example, W. B. Grayson, "Malaria Control in Arkansas, 1933," *South Med J* 27 (1934): 652; "Malaria Incidence 1934–5," *South Med J* 28 (1935): 765; F. C. Dugan, "Malaria Control in Kentucky," *Bull Dept Health, Comm Ky* 9 (1937): 257–59.

27. M. R. Cowper, "Malaria Control and Minor Drainage by Open Ditches," *Health Bull (NC)* 48 (Jul. 1933): 8–10.

28. George E. Riley and Nelson Rector, "Experience with Minor Drainage in Relation to Malaria Rates in Some Mississippi Delta Counties," *South Med J* 30 (1937): 862–66.

29. C. C. Dauer and E. C. Faust, "Malaria Mortality," *South Med J* 30 (1937): 939–43.

30. Ernest Carroll Faust, "Malaria Mortality in the Southern U.S. for the Year 1936," *South Med J* 31 (1938): 816–18; W. V. King, "Historical Developments and Progress in Our Knowledge of Malaria Control," *South Med J* 31 (1938): 797–802; J. B. Pomerance, "Brief Remarks on Malaria," *J Florida Med Assoc* 26 (1939): 341–43.

31. Bispham, "Malaria," 848, 850.

32. Cited in T. J. Woofter, Jr., and A. E. Fisher, *The Plantation South Today* (Washington, D.C.: U.S. Government Printing Office, 1940), 17.

33. William C. Holley et al., *The Plantation South 1934–1937* (Washington, D.C.: U. S. Government Printing Office, 1940), 61.

34. Carl V. Reynolds to George W. Coan, Jr., Jun. 9, 1937, reprinted in *North Carolina WPA: Its Story* 2, no.7 (1937).

35. *Boondoggling. The Story of the "$25,000" Memphis Dog House and Other Stories* (Washington: Record, 1936). This pamphlet is a Democratic publication that first gives the Republican caricature of various WPA projects, then defends them with "the true story."

36. H. L. Mencken, "Three Years of Dr. Roosevelt" (1936), reprinted in Leuchtenburg, *The New Deal: A Documentary History*, 200–201.

37. *Biennial Rep Tenn Dept Public Health, 1933–35*, 75–85.

38. C. W. Garrison, "Malaria Control in Arkansas in 1932," *South Med J* 26 (1933): 469–70.

39. *Biennial Rep Tenn Dept Public Health, 1933–35*, 75–82.

40. Nelson H. Rector, "Drainage and Filling Methods for Malaria and Malaria Control," in Moulton, ed., *Symposium on Human Malaria*, 315–23, at 315.

41. S. W. Simmons, "Progress in the Development of Malaria Control Techniques," *J Nat Malaria Soc* 5 (1946): 157–63, at 162. See also Justin Andrews,

"What's Happening to Malaria in the USA?" *Am J Public Health* 38 (1948): 931–42.

42.  George B. Tindall, *The Emergence of the New South: 1913–1945* (Baton Rouge: Louisiana State University Press, 1967), 447. See also Michael J. McDonald and John Muldowny, *TVA and the Dispossessed* (Knoxville: University of Tennessee Press, 1982), and Walter L. Creese, *TVA's Public Planning: The Vision, The Reality* (Knoxville: University of Tennessee Press, 1990).

43.  George Bradley, "A Review of Malaria Control and Eradication in the United States," *Mosq News* 26 (1966): 462–70, at 464.

44.  [W. G. Stromquist], "Malaria and Impounded Waters," in *Malaria Control for Engineers: Report of the National Malaria Committee.* (Washington: USPHS, 1936), 23–31, 30–31.

45.  Tindall, *Emergence,* 452.

46.  Robert Briggs Watson and Margaret E. Rice, "Some Epidemiological Characteristics of Malaria in North Alabama as Determined by Data Collected over the Twenty-year Period 1923–1942," *Am J Hyg* 40 (1944): 199–208; Robert Briggs Watson and Margaret E. Rice, "Notes on the Morbidity of Naturally Occurring Malaria," *J Nat Malaria Soc* 5 (1946): 7–12; Robert Briggs Watson, Calvin C. Kiker, and Archie Hess, "A Review of Malaria Studies and Control in the Tennessee Valley in 1945," *J Nat Malaria Soc* 5 (1946): 193–203; and Calvin C. Kiker, Charles D. Fairer, and Paul N. Flanary, "Further Observations on Airplane Dusting for *Anopheles* Larvae Control," *South Med J* 31 (1938): 808–13. E. Harold Hinman and H. S. Hurlbut, "A Study of Winter Activities and Hibernation of Anopheles Quadrimaculatus in the Tennessee Valley," *Am J Trop Med* 20 (1940): 431–46; T. F. Hall and A. D. Hess, "Plant Control Studies in Tennessee Valley Reservoirs," *J Nat Malaria Soc* 9 (1950): 153–72; and A. D. Hess and R. L. Crowell, "Seasonal History of *Anopheles quadrimaculatus* in the Tennessee Valley," *J Nat Malaria Soc* 8 (1949): 159–70.

47.  Mary Humphreys, interview, Nov. 7, 1993.

48.  Kiker, Fairer, and Flanary, "Further Observations," 808–13; C. W. Krusé and R. L. Metcalf, "An Analysis of the Design and Performance of Airplane Exhaust Generators for the Production of DDT Aerosols for the Control of *Anopheles Quadrimaculatus,*" *Public Health Rep* 61 (1946): 1171–84.

49.  F. E. Gartrell, "Statement of Progress of Kentucky Reservoir Malaria Control Program," *J Nat Malaria Soc* 4 (1945): 63–65; and F. E. Gartrell and A. H. Johnson, "A Study to Evaluate Malaria Control Projects of Kentucky Reservoir in Terms of Collateral Uses and Socio-economic Benefits," *J Nat Malaria Soc* 9 (1950): 259–67.

50.  Watson and Rice, "Some Epidemiological Characteristics."

51.  Walter B. Edgar, *History of Santee-Cooper 1934–1984* (Columbia: R. L. Bryan, 1984). This brief and copiously illustrated history was funded by the South Carolina Public Service Authority and makes no mention of the malaria generated by the project.

52.  Edgar, *History of Santee-Cooper,* 10. On the standard methods for creating malaria-free impounded water projects, see E. Harold Hinman, "The Manage-

ment of Water for Malaria Control," in Moulton, ed., *Symposium on Human Malaria*, 324–32.

53.    Henry A. Johnson, "Inspection of the Santee and Pinopolis Reservoirs of the South Carolina Public Service Authority Relative to the Hazards from Malaria," inspection made Sept. 11–17, 1944, Folder named "1850-Santee Cooper Survey," Central Files Correspondence, 1942–51, Box 98, Record Group 444, CDCA.

54.    "A Malaria Survey of the Santee-Cooper Impoundment," *Malaria Control in War Areas Field Bull*, June 1945; *Malaria Control in War Areas, 1944–45*, 52–55.

55.    Memo from R. F. Reider to A. G. Gilliam, Oct. 6, 1944, in Folder named "Malaria Field Studies (Manning, S.C.)," Center Director General Files, Box 6, Record Group 444, CDCA.

56.    "A Malaria Survey of the Santee-Cooper Impoundment," *Malaria Control in War Areas Field Bull*, June 1945; *Malaria Control in War Areas, 1944–45*, 52–55.

57.    Uncatalogued papers related to malaria campaigns of the North Carolina State Board of Health, Public Health Pest Management Section, Division of Environmental Health, North Carolina Department of Environment, Health and Natural Resources, Raleigh, N.C.

58.    "A Malaria Survey of the Santee-Cooper Impoundment," *Malaria Control in War Areas Field Bull*, June 1945; W. G. Smillie, "Studies of an Epidemic of Malaria at the Gantt Impounded Area, Covington Co., Alabama," *Am J Hyg* 7 (1927): 40–72.

59.    Oliver Wendell Holmes, "Dissertation on Intermittent Fevers in New England," *Boylston Prize Dissertations for the Years 1836 and 1837* (Boston: Charles C. Little and James Brown, 1838).

60.    Gilbert C. Fite, *Cotton Fields No More: Southern Agriculture 1865–1980* (Lexington: University Press of Kentucky, 1984): 120–62.

61.    Ibid., 56–77. See also Roger Biles, "The Urban South in the Great Depression," *J South Hist* 56 (1990): 71–100.

62.    Gunnar Myrdal, *An American Dilemma: The Negro Problem and Modern Democracy*, 2 vols. (New York: Harper and Brothers, 1944), 1: 46, 74.

63.    Jack T. Kirby, *Rural Worlds Lost: The American South 1920–1960*. (Baton Rouge and London: Louisiana State University Press, 1987), xv.

64.    Nicholas Lemann, *The Promised Land: The Great Black Migration and How It Changed America* (New York: Random House, 1991); James R. Grossman, *Land of Hope: Chicago, Black Southerners, and the Great Migration* (Chicago: University of Chicago Press, 1989); and Neil Fligstein, *Going North: Migration of Blacks and Whites from the South, 1900–1950* (New York: Academic Press, 1981).

65.    M. A. Barber, "Malaria in the Prairie Rice Regions of Louisiana and Arkansas," *Public Health Rep* 41 (1926): 2527–49, at 2546.

66.    Andrews, "What's Happening to Malaria," 931–42.

1. Sheila M. Rothman, *Living in the Shadow of Death: Tuberculosis and the Social Experience of Illness in American History* (New York: Basic Books, 1994).

2. Christopher Feudtner, "The Want of Control: Ideas, Innovations, and Ideals in the Modern Management of Diabetes Mellitus," *Bull Hist Med* 69 (1995): 66–90.

3. On the Federal Writers' Project, see Monty Noam Penkower, *The Federal Writers' Project: A Study in Government Patronage of the Arts* (Urbana: University of Illinois Press, 1977); C. Vann Woodward, "History from Slave Sources," *Am Hist Rev* 79 (1974): 470–81; Jeutonne P. Brewer, *The Federal Writers' Project: A Bibliography* (Metuchen, N.J.: Scarecrow Press, 1994); and Jerre Mangione, *The Dream and the Deal: The Federal Writers' Project, 1935–43* (Boston: Little, Brown & Co., 1972).

4. Charles S. Johnson, *Shadow of the Plantation* (Chicago: University of Chicago Press, 1934).

5. Josie Fleming, narrative, FWP-SHC. On midwives in the South, see Margaret Charles Smith and Linda Janet Holmes, *Listen to Me Good: The Life Story of an Alabama Midwife* (Columbus: Ohio State University Press, 1996), and Gertrude Jacinda Fraser, *African American Midwifery in the South: Dialogues of Birth, Race, and Memory* (Cambridge, Mass.: Harvard University Press, 1998).

6. Lula Coleman, narrative in George Rawick, ed., *The American Slave: A Composite Autobiography,* supp., ser. 1, vol. 7, Mississippi Narratives, pt. 2 (Westport, Conn.: Greenwood Press, 1977), 434. These volumes contain facsimile reproductions of the FWP slave interview typescripts from the late 1930s.

7. Johnson, *Shadow* , 192. Johnson frequently reprinted strings of quotations from his interviews.

8. Quoted in ibid., 193–95.

9. Charles Pollard, quoted in James H. Jones, *Bad Blood: The Tuskegee Syphilis Experiment,* 2d ed. (New York: Free Press, 1993), 6–7.

10. Martha Cox, narrative in Rawick, ed., *American Slave,* supp., ser. 1, vol. 11, North Carolina and South Carolina Narratives, 105.

11. Ella Small, narrative in Rawick, ed., *American Slave,* supp., ser. 1, vol. 11, North Carolina and South Carolina Narratives, 287.

12. Becky Clayton, narrative in James Seay Brown, Jr., ed., *Up before Daylight: Life Histories from the Alabama Writer's Project, 1938–1939* (University: University of Alabama Press, 1982), 163.

13. Quoted in Johnson, *Shadow,* 193.

14. The classic essay on this phenomenon is Susan Sontag, *Illness as Metaphor and AIDS and Its Metaphors* (New York: Anchor Books, 1989).

15. Fannie Icord, narrative, FWP-SHC.

16. Josie Fleming, narrative, FWP-SHC.

17. Liza Howard, quoted in Henry Howard, narrative, FWP-SHC.

18. Mary Staton Jones, narrative, FWP-SHC.

19. D. E. Cadwallader and F. J. Wilson, "Folklore Medicine among Georgia's Piedmont Negroes after the Civil War," *Georgia Hist Q* 49 (1965): 217–27. Also useful is John K. Crellin and Jane Philpott, *A Reference Guide to Medicinal Plants: Herbal Medicine Past and Present* (1989; reprint Durham, N.C.: Duke University Press, 1997).

20. Lula Coleman, narrative, in Rawick, ed., *American Slave,* supp., ser. 1, vol. 7, Mississippi Narratives, pt. 2, 432.

21. Mrs. Jim Shelton, narrative, FWP-SHC.

22. Tank Valentine Daughtry, narrative, FWP-SHC.

23. George White, narrative, in Charles L. Perdue, Thomas F. Barden, and Robert K. Phillips, eds., *Weevils in the Wheat: Interviews with Virginia Ex-Slaves* (Charlottesville: University of Virginia Press, 1976), 310.

24. Cadwallader and Wilson, "Folklore Medicine."

25. For further information, see Elliott J. Gorn, "Folk Beliefs of the Slave Community," in Ronald L. Numbers and Todd L. Savitt, eds., *Science and Medicine in the Old South* (Baton Rouge: Louisiana State University Press, 1989), 295–326.

26. Patsy Moses, narrative, in James Mellon, ed., *Bullwhip Days: The Slaves Remember: An Oral History* (New York: Avon Books, 1988), 96.

27. Uncle Shang Harris, narrative, in Rawick, ed., *American Slave,* vol. 12, Georgia Narratives, pt. 2, 123.

28. Estella Jones, narrative, in Mellon, ed., *Bullwhip Days,* 98.

29. Emmaline Heard, narrative, in Rawick, ed., *American Slave,* vol. 12, Georgia Narratives, pt. 2, 157–58.

30. Mary DeRoy, narrative, FWP-SHC.

31. Henry Baysmore, narrative, FWP-SHC.

32. Newton Owen, narrative, FWP-SHC; William Adams, narrative, in Mellon, ed., *Bullwhip Days,* 74.

33. No name, narrative titled "Outcast in the World," FWP-SHC.

34. Committee on the Costs of Medical Care, *Medical Care for the American People. The Final Report of the Committee on the Costs of Medical Care* (Chicago: University of Chicago Press, 1932), 29.

35. Johnson, *Shadow,* 192; Fred Poinsette, narrative, in Rawick, ed., *American Slave,* supp., ser. 1, vol. 11, North Carolina and South Carolina narratives, 272.

36. Lula and Allison Sizemore, narrative, FWP-SHC.

37. George and Sally Dobbin, narrative, in W. T. Couch, ed., *These Are Our Lives, as Told by the People and Written by Members of the Federal Writers' Project of the Works Progress Administration* (Chapel Hill: University of North Carolina Press, 1939), 208–09.

38. Johnson, *Shadow,* 196.

39. Lewis Little, narrative, FWP-SHC.

40.   Dona Balmer, narrative, FWP-SHC.

41.   Archie Booker, narrative, in Perdue, ed., *Weevils,* 54.

42.   Jennie Rowe, narrative, FWP-SHC.

43.   Mary Bloomberg, narrative, FWP-SHC.

44.   No name, narrative titled "When Spring Comes," FWP-SHC.

45.   James Hillyer, narrative, FWP-SHC.

46.   Roy and Fannie Woods, narrative, FWP-SHC.

47.   Will Conner, narrative, FWP-SHC.

48.   Edward H. Beardsley, *A History of Neglect: Health Care for Blacks and Mill Workers in the Twentieth-Century South* (Knoxville: University of Tennessee Press, 1987).

49.   Walter Raleigh Parker, narrative, FWP-SHC.

50.   Johnnie Fence, narrative, in Brown, ed., *Up before Daylight,* 100–1.

51.   Rosa Hanks, narrative, in Brown, ed., *Up before Daylight,* 211.

52.   Mandy Johnson, narrative, FWP-SHC.

53.   J. B. Fearing, narrative, FWP-SHC.

54.   Emaline, narrative, in Tom E. Terrill and Jerold Hirsch, eds., *Such as Us: Southern Voices of the Thirties* (Chapel Hill: University of North Carolina Press, 1979), 80.

55.   Mr. and Mrs. Elmer Ray, narrative, FWP-SHC.

56.   Nannie Hawkins, narrative, FWP-SHC.

57.   Kate Brumby, narrative, in Couch, ed., *These Are Our Lives,* 157.

58.   John Vinson, narrative, FWP-SHC.

59.   Sarah Myers, narrative, FWP-SHC.

60.   George Briggs, narrative, in Rawick, ed., *American Slave,* supp., ser. 1, vol. 11, North Carolina and South Carolina narratives, 74.

61.   No name, narrative titled "They Would Tie You up and Whip You," in Ophelia Settle Egypt, J. Masouka, and Charles S. Johnson, *Unwritten History of Slavery* (1945); reprint in Rawick, ed., *American Slave,* vol. 18, 248.

62.   Valentine and Delbert Hunter, narrative, FWP-SHC.

63.   James Lucas, narrative, in Rawick, ed., *American Slave,* supp., ser. 1, vol. 8, Mississippi narratives, 1346.

64.   Cornelius Garner, narrative, in Perdue, ed., *Weevils,* 104.

65.   Ennion G. Williams, "Rural Malaria Control with the County as the Unit," *South Med J* 15 (1922): 362–68, at 362–63.

66.   Oscar Dowling, *Health Conditions in Louisiana* (n.p., ca.1911).

67.   Margaret Humphreys, *Yellow Fever and the South* (1992; reprint, Baltimore: Johns Hopkins University Press, 1998), 164.

68.   W. C. Johnson, "Our Malaria Campaign," *South Med J* 11 (1918): 572–74, at 573.

69. D. F. Ashton, "Malaria Control: A Cooperative Venture," *Health Bull (NC)* 58, no. 19 (Oct. 1943): 9–11, at 9.

70. Ashton, "Malaria Control," 9.

71. William Batts, narrative, FWP-SHC.

72. Fannie Icord, narrative, FWP-SHC.

73. Emaline, narrative, in Terrill and Hirsch, eds., *Such as Us,* 80–81.

74. John Ettling, *The Germ of Laziness: Rockefeller Philanthropy and Public Health in the New South* (Cambridge, Mass.: Harvard University Press, 1981), 170.

75. C. C. Bass, "Difficulties and Errors before and after Anti-malaria Campaigns," *South Med J* 15 (1922): 339–43, at 339.

76. Kenneth F. Maxcy, "Epidemiological Principles Affecting the Distribution of Malaria in Southern United States," *Public Health Rep* 39 (1924): 1113–27, at 1119.

77. L. D. Fricks, "Malaria Control in the United States: Retrospect and Prospect," *South Med J* 17 (1924): 578–82, at 582.

78. "Contest Opens, February 9th," 1920 poster of the North Carolina Landowners Association, in uncatalogued papers related to malaria campaigns of the North Carolina State Board of Health, Public Health Pest Management Section, Division of Environmental Health, North Carolina Department of Environment, Health and Natural Resources, Raleigh, N.C.

79. M. A. Fort, "Malaria Control Activities in Georgia," *South Med J* 18 (1925): 469–70, at 470.

80. Zora Neale Hurston, *Mules and Men* (1935; reprint New York: HarperPerennial, 1990), 136–37.

81. Rosa Faison, narrative, FWP-SHC.

82. Anonymous, narrative, Folder 413a, FWP-SHC. "RRR" was a chill tonic that contained quinine.

83. "Free Negro," in Egypt, Masouka, and Johnson, *Unwritten History of Slavery,* reprint in Rawick, ed., *American Slave,* 313.

84. George Briggs, narrative, in Rawick, ed., *American Slave,* supp. 1, ser. 1, vol. 11, North Carolina and South Carolina narratives, 73.

85. Raymond Barbour, narrative, FWP-SHC; see also Lula Rousseau, narrative, FWP-SHC.

86. Mamie Wilson, narrative, FWP-SHC.

87. Sam the Turpentine Chopper, narrative, FWP-SHC.

88. Bob and Christine Curtis, narrative, FWP-SHC.

89. Cato, narrative, in B. A. Botkin, ed., *Lay My Burden Down: A Folk History of Slavery* (Chicago: University of Chicago Press, 1945), 83–89, at 86.

90. Leathy Lightsey, narrative, FWP-SHC.

91. George Fallow, narrative, in Terrill and Hirsch, eds., *Such as Us,* 205–18, at 216–17.

92. Christine and Bob Curtis, narrative, FWP-SHC.

93. Robert S. Desowitz, *Who Gave Pinta to the Santa Maria? Torrid Diseases in a Temperate World* (New York: W. W. Norton, 1997), 194.

94. Pattie Debrow, narrative, FWP-SHC.

95. Thomas Cole, narrative, in Mellon, ed., *Bullwhip Days,* 55–72, at 71.

96. Photographs, Records of the USPHS, Record Group 90, NACP.

CHAPTER SEVEN: DENOUEMENT

1. "Civilian Control: Possibility of Malaria Endemicity Much Less than in 1945–47," *Public Health Rep* 67 (1952): 179.

2. Useful background histories of the U. S. Health Service are Ralph Chester Williams, *The United States Public Health Service, 1798–1950* (Washington: Commissioned Officers Association of the U. S. Public Health Service, 1951); and Fitzhugh Mullan, *Plagues and Politics: The Story of the United States Public Health Service* (New York: Basic Books, 1989). On the CDC itself, see Elizabeth W. Etheridge, *Sentinel for Health: A History of the Centers for Disease Control* (Berkeley: University of California Press, 1992).

3. Ernest Carroll Faust, "Certain Factors in the Epidemiology of Malaria in the Southern United States," *N Orl Med Surg J* 89 (1936–37): 692–94; Ernest Carroll Faust, "Distribution of Malaria in North America, Central America, and the West Indies," in Forest Ray Moulton, ed., *A Symposium on Human Malaria with Special Reference to North America and the Caribbean Region* (Washington: American Association for the Advancement of Science, 1941), 8–18; W. N. Bispham, "Malaria in the Southern States," *South Med J* 32 (1939): 848–51, at 848, 850.

4. *Malaria Control in War Areas, 1945–46,* 63–70; *Biennial Rep Tenn Dept Public Health 1943–45,* 67.

5. Etheridge, *Sentinel for Health,* 34.

6. Ernest Carroll Faust and Lois DeBakey, "Malaria Mortality in the Southern United States for the Year 1940, with Supplementary Data on Malaria in Other States," *J Nat Malaria Soc* 1 (1941): 125–31, at 125.

7. Louis L. Williams, "The Anti-malaria Program in North America," in Moulton, ed., *Symposium on Human Malaria,* 365–70, at 366; *Malaria Control in War Areas, 1942–43,* cover and p. 1; *Malaria Control in War Areas, 1943–44,* 7.

8. Justin Andrews and Jean S. Grant, "Experience in the United States," in Ebbe Hoff, ed., *Preventive Medicine in World War II* (Washington: Office of the Surgeon General, 1963), vol. 6, 61–112, at 61–62.

9. *Malaria Control in War Areas, 1943–44,* 2.

10. Paul F. Russell, "A Lively Corpse," *Trop Med News* 5 (June 1948): 25. See also Ernest Carroll Faust, "Clinical and Public Health Aspects of Malaria in the United States from an Historical Perspective," *Am J Trop Med* 25 (1945): 185–201, at 192, and Erwin Ackerknecht, *Malaria in the Upper Mississippi Valley, 1760–1900* (Baltimore: Johns Hopkins University Press, 1945), 1.

11. On the "swine flu" episode, see June E. Osborn, ed., *History, Science and Politics: Influenza in America, 1918–1976* (New York: Prodist, 1977), and Richard

Neustadt and Harvey Fineberg, *The Epidemic That Never Was: Policy Making and the Swine Flu Scare* (New York: Vintage Books, 1983).

12.      Paul F. Russell, *Man's Mastery of Malaria* (London: Oxford University Press, 1955), 117.

13.      See Albert E. Cowdrey, *Fighting for Life: American Military Medicine in World War II* (New York: Free Press, 1994), and Mary Ellen Condon-Rall, "The Role of the U.S. Army in the Fight against Malaria, 1940–1944," *War Soc* 13 (1995): 91–111.

14.      James Phinney Baxter, *Scientists against Time* (Boston: Little, Brown & Co., 1946), 299–320, 360–76.

15.      James Stevens Simmons, "Global Malaria," *N Engl J Med* 229 (1943): 605–10; and Omar J. Brown, "The Malaria Control Program of the Navy," *J Nat Malaria Soc* 3 (1944): 15–18.

16.      Thomas A. Hart, "The Army's War against Malaria," *Scientific Monthly* (1946), 421–22, at 421.

17.      Brown, "Malaria Control," 18.

18.      See Chapter 4, note 6. This film was discussed in a *Time* magazine article of June 14, 1943.

19.      *Malaria Control in War Areas, 1943–43,* 5.

20.      Charles M. White et al., "Malaria Control in the United States," *J Nat Malaria Soc* 4 (1945): 52–55.

21.      Andrews and Grant, "Experience," 83–90.

22.      *Malaria Control in War Areas, 1944–45* (Washington: U.S. Public Health Service, 1945), 1–2; and Stanley Freeborn, "The Malaria Control Program of the United States Public Health Service among Civilians in Extra-Military Areas," *J Nat Malaria Soc* 3 (1944): 19–23.

23.      Martin D. Young et al., "Studies on Imported Malarias. 10. An Evaluation of the Foreign Malarias Introduced into the United States by Returning Troops," *J Nat Malaria Soc* 7 (1948): 171–85.

24.      *Congressional Record,* 78th Cong., 2nd sess., 6486 (June 22, 1944). Similar comments were made in the House; see ibid., 4796 (May 22, 1944). The text of the law is found in ibid., 4800–4811 (May 22, 1944), and was published in *Laws Relating to the United States Public Health Service* (Washington: U.S. Public Health Service, 1947).

25.      This attitude did not change during the war, as successive MCWA reports indicate. See *Malaria Control in War Areas, 1942–43,* 10; *Malaria Control in War Areas, 1943–44,* 12–16; and *Malaria Control in War Areas, 1944–45,* 8.

26.      Uncatalogued papers related to malaria campaigns of the North Carolina State Board of Health, Public Health Pest Management Section, Division of Environmental Health, North Carolina Department of Environment, Health, and Natural Resources, Raleigh, N.C.

27.      Freeborn, "Malaria Control," 21.

28.      See the MCWA annual reports, and Andrews and Grant, "Experience."

29. John L. Porter (assistant director, Division of Public Health Engineering, Louisiana) to Mark Hollis (MCWA official), Aug. 23, 1944, in Box 97, "1850-Louisiana," Central Files—Correspondence, Communicable Disease Center Papers, Record Group 442, CDCA.

30. G. H. Bradley to John L. Porter, Aug. 26, 1944, ibid.

31. Elliott H. Pennell (statistician of the states relation division of MCWA) to Trawick H. Stubbs, Dec. 10, 1942, Box 527, "Malaria," General Classified Records, Group IX—General Files 1936-1944, Records of the USPHS, Record Group 90, NACP.

32. Due to Williams's ill health, the assistant surgeon general, J. W. Mountin, presented and published his proposal. See J. W. Mountin, "A Program for the Eradication of Malaria from Continental United States," *J Nat Malaria Soc* 3 (1944): 69-73, and Stanley Freeborn, "Problems Created by Returning Malaria Carriers," *Public Health Rep* 59 (1944): 357-63, at 358-59.

33. William S. Boyd et. al., "Educational Activities as Related to the Extended Malaria Control Program: A Progress Report," *J Nat Malaria Soc* 5 (1946): 245-51, at 245.

34. *Malaria Control in War Areas, 1945-46,* viii.

35. Baxter, *Scientists,* 375; Marshall Barber, *A Malariologist in Many Lands* (Lawrence: University of Kansas Press, 1946), 24.

36. Meeting of Advisory Committee, Malaria Control Field Station, Jan. 8, 1952, in Box 7, "Newton Field Station," Center Director General Files, Record group 442, CDCA.

37. Etheridge, *Sentinel,* 1-17.

38. Justin Andrews and Wesley E. Gilbertson, "Blueprint for Malaria Eradication in the United States," *CDC Bull* (April, May, June 1948): 1-3, at 1.

39. MCWA officials were not alone in seeking to parlay the war's generation of "emergency funding" and institutional growth into peacetime expansion. See Michael Aaron Dennis, "'Our First Line of Defense': Two University Laboratories in the Postwar American State," *Isis* 85 (1994): 427-55, for similar challenges faced by defense research laboratories.

40. E. F. Knipling, "The Development and Use of DDT for the Control of Mosquitoes," *J Nat Malaria Soc* 4 (1945): 77-92; Oliver R. McCoy, "War Department Provisions for Malaria Control," in Hoff, ed., *Preventive Medicine in World War II,* 11-59, at 42-48. The best secondary account of DDT's development is Thomas R. Dunlap, *DDT: Scientists, Citizens and Public Policy* (Princeton, N.J.: Princeton University Press, 1981). See also John H. Perkins, "Reshaping Technology in Wartime: The Effect of Military Goals on Entomological Research and Insect-Control Practices," *Technology and Culture* 19 (1978): 169-86. On insecticides available before World War II, see James Whorton, *Before Silent Spring: Pesticides and Public Health in Pre-DDT America* (Princeton, N.J.: Princeton University Press, 1974).

41. McCoy, "War Department," 40.

42. Russell, "The United States and Malaria," 635-36; Baxter, *Scientists,* 360-76; and *Malaria Control in War Areas, 1943-44,* 21.

43. Dunlap, *DDT,* 62. On the typhus control problem in World War II, see Albert E. Cowdrey, *War and Healing: Stanhope Bayne-Jones and the Maturing of American Medicine* (Baton Rouge: Louisiana State University Press, 1992), 151–59.

44. "Taking Stock of DDT," *Am J Public Health* 36 (1946): 657–58, at 658.

45. Paul F. Russell, "Introduction," in Hoff, ed., *Preventive Medicine in World War II,* 1–10, at 10. On the technical problems involved in atomizing DDT and expelling it from a plane, and on its use in domestic operations, see C. W. Krusé and R. L. Metcalf, "An Analysis of the Design and Performance of Airplane Exhaust Generators for the Production of DDT Aerosols for the Control of Anopheles quadrimaculatus," *Public Health Rep* 61 (1946): 1171–84.

46. "Taking Stock," 657; *Malaria Control in War Areas, 1945–46;* and Dunlap, *DDT,* 3.

47. Justin Andrews, "Advancing Frontiers in Insect Vector Control," *Am J Public Health* 40 (1950): 409–16, at 409.

48. Lois Mattox Miller, "What You Should Know about DDT," *Reader's Digest,* 47 (1945): 84–86, at 84 (reprinted from the *Baltimore Sunday Sun,* date unknown).

49. *Malaria Control in War Areas, 1944–45,* 21–23, 40–41.

50. Edmund P. Russell, "'Speaking of Annihilation:' Mobilizing for War against Human and Insect Enemies, 1914–1945," *J Am Hist* 82 (1996): 1505–29.

51. *Malaria Control in War Areas, 1944–45,* 21.

52. Jens A. Jensen, "The DDT Residual Spraying Program for Malaria Control in North Carolina," *Health Bull (NC)* 60 (Oct. 1945): 12–14; and Boyd, "Educational Activities," 250.

53. Sidney Margolis, "DDT Is No Cure-All," *Colliers* 116 (Nov. 17, 1945): 27, 57, at 27.

54. Andrews and Gilbertson, "Blueprint." Each *CDC Bulletin* included tables of houses sprayed, man-hours expended, and quantities of DDT used.

55. Leon J. Warshaw, *Malaria: The Biography of a Killer* (New York: Rinehart & Co., 1949), 152.

56. James Stevens Simmons, "American Mobilization for the Conquest of Malaria in the United States," *J Nat Malaria Soc* 3 (1944): 7–10, at 10.

57. *Malaria Control in War Areas, 1944–45,* 14–15.

58. Frederick L. Knowles and Clinton S. Smith, "DDT Residual House Spray—A Method of Malaria Control in Rural Areas," *Public Health Rep* 60 (1945): 1274–79; F. Earle Lyman, "Results of the Residual DDT Spray Program against Malaria Mosquitoes, 1945–1949," *CDC Bull* (Jan. 1950), 10–13.

59. Andrews and Grant, "Experience," 91.

60. George H. Bradley and Melvin H. Goodwin, Jr., "Malaria Observation Stations of the Public Health Service," *J Nat Malaria Soc* 8 (1949): 181–91, at 181.

61. Andrews, "Malaria Eradication," 1405.

62. Paul F. Russell, "Some Epidemiological Aspects of Malaria Control with Reference to DDT," *J Nat Malaria Soc* 10 (1951): 257–65, at 259; Justin M. Andrews, "Nationwide Malaria Eradication Projects in the Americas: The Eradication Program in the U.S.A.," *J Nat Malaria Soc* 10 (1951): 99–121, at 113.

63. Alexander D. Langmuir, MD (chief of epidemiology branch, CDC) to Dr. J. M. Andrews, Oct. 8, 1952, in Box 2, "Others," Center Director General Files, Record Group 442, CDCA.

64. *Malaria Control in War Areas, 1944–45,* 50–55.

65. Quoted in . . . *For the Nation's Health: Orientation and Training Manual, Communicable Disease Center* (Atlanta: Communicable Disease Center, 1948), xii, 47–48.

66. Christine Beadle and Stephen L. Hoffman, "History of Malaria in the United States Naval Forces at War: World War I through the Vietnam Conflict," *Clin Infect Dis* 16 (1993): 320–29; "Malaria Surveillance—United States, 1994," supp., *Morb Mort Wkly Rep* 46 (Oct. 17, 1997); and Peter J. Weina, "From Atabrine in World War II to Mefloquine in Somalia: The Role of Education in Preventive Medicine," *Mil Med* 163 (1998): 635–36.

67. See Gordon Harrison, *Mosquitoes, Malaria and Man: A History of the Hostilities since 1880* (New York: E. P. Dutton, 1978), 228–38, and Leonard Jan Bruce-Chwatt and Julian de Zulueta, *The Rise and Fall of Malaria in Europe: A Historico-Epidemiological Study* (Oxford: Oxford University Press, 1980), 167–73.

68. Russell et al., *Practical Malariology* (1963), 21–22.

69. Socrates Litsios, *The Tomorrow of Malaria* (Wellington, New Zealand: Pacific Press, 1996), 92–105.

70. Robert S. Desowitz, *The Malaria Capers: More Tales of Parasites and People, Research and Reality* (New York: W. W. Norton, 1991); and David J. Wyler, "Malaria—Resurgence, Resistance, and Research," *N Engl J Med* 308 (1983): 875–78, 934–40.

71. Russell, "The United States and Malaria," 643, 648.

72. Ibid., 650.

73. Paul F. Russell, "Malaria and Its Influence on World Health," *Bull N Y Acad Med* 19 (1943): 599–630, at 628.

# Note on Sources

My initial interest in the history of malaria was sparked by reading Erwin Ackerknecht's *Malaria in the Upper Mississippi Valley, 1760–1900* (Baltimore: Johns Hopkins University Press, 1945), and that remains the proper starting point for the student of malaria's history in the United States. Ackerknecht's approach to understanding the causation of malaria and the reasons for its persistence within one region has influenced my own from the beginning of this project. Ackerknecht in turn mined the works of some of the best malariologists of his day—Lewis Hackett, Mark Boyd, Ernst Carroll Faust, and M. A. Barber, to name a few—in manufacturing his sophisticated approach to malaria in nineteenth-century America. Through reading Ackerknecht and his sources, I came to understand the complex web of socioeconomic as well as biological influences that make up the etiological nexus of malaria. I follow Ackerknecht in denying that "malaria . . . [is] a purely social disease," while at the same time concluding with him that "economic factors are so closely interwoven with the possibilities of anopheline transmission, that any study of malaria has to include the study of such social phenomena" (p. 66). His influence can be seen on most every page of this work.

This book also grew out of my prior research on yellow fever, in *Yellow Fever and the South* (1992; reprint Baltimore: Johns Hopkins University Press, 1998). Both yellow fever and malaria are tropical diseases only temporarily at home in the United States, both are transmitted by mosquitoes, and both came ultimately to stigmatize the American South as particularly diseased. The segue from yellow fever, which disappeared in 1905, to malaria, whose focused attack began only in the next decade, flowed easily.

Aside from Ackerknecht's seminal work, publications on the history of malaria in the United States are rather scarce. Articles by Mark Boyd and Ernst Carroll Faust in the 1940s, and by Paul Russell in 1968, were the principal source of John Duffy's brief account of malaria published in 1988, "The Impact of Malaria on the South," in Todd L. Savitt and James Harvey Young, eds., *Disease and Distinctiveness in the American South* (Knoxville: University of Tennessee Press, 1988): 29–54. See Ernest Carroll Faust, "Clinical and Public Health Aspects of Malaria in the United States from an Historical Perspective," *Am J Trop Med* 25 (1945): 185–201; Mark F. Boyd, "An Historical Sketch of the Prevalence of Malaria in North America," *Am J Trop Med* 21 (1941): 223-244; and Paul F. Russell, "The United States and Malaria: Debits and Credits," *Bull N Y Acad Med* 44 (1968): 623–53. A master's thesis by James Rodney Young is also useful for its detailed account of the Rockefeller demonstration projects: *Malaria in the South, 1900–1930* (Ann Arbor: University Microfilms, 1972).

More has been written on the history of malaria in general. Gordon Harrison's *Mosquitoes, Malaria and Man: A History of the Hostilities since 1880* (New York: E. P. Dutton, 1978) remains the best overall account, while Leonard Jan Bruce-Chwatt and Julian de Zulveta cover the story for Europe in *The Rise and Fall of Malaria in Europe: A Historico-epidemiological Study* (Oxford: Oxford University Press, 1980). Mary Dobson's work on early modern England is a model for dissecting the history of a disease so closely tied to geography, economy, and demographic factors: *Contours of Death and Disease in Early Modern England* (Cambridge: Cambridge University Press, 1997).

Several archives offer particularly rich source material for the history of malaria in the United States. The papers of the U.S. Public Health Service are now housed in the National Archives branch at College Park, Maryland (Record Group 90). The Rockefeller Archives in Sleepy Hollow, New York, contain reports concerning the malaria research done in the South from 1916 to 1940, including the initial demonstration projects after World War I and the diaries of Mark Boyd while at work in Tallahassee. The National Archives branch at East Point, Georgia (a suburb of Atlanta), houses the papers of the Malaria Control in War Areas agency and the early years of the CDC. The unpublished Federal Writers' Project manuscript narratives used in this book are found in the University of North Carolina at Chapel Hill's Southern Historical Collection. Material on the North Carolina malaria campaigns of the 1930s and 1940s came from boxes stored in the office of the state's medical entomologist, Dr. Barry Engber.

After working on the nineteenth century when studying yellow fever, the sheer abundance of twentieth-century publications on malaria was a bit daunting. Several journals are particularly rich sources of articles on malaria work in the United States. Beginning in the early twentieth century, the Southern Medical Association held an annual symposium on malaria, and it was published in the organization's organ, the *Southern Medical Journal*. This yearly section branched off into a different journal and organization in 1941, becoming the *Journal of the National Malaria Society*, which in turn merged with the *American Journal of Tropical Medicine* in 1952. The *American Journal of Public Health* also published articles on malaria. Throughout the twentieth century the *Public Health Reports* of the U. S. Public Health Service documented malaria work in the South, while during World War II the Malaria Control in War Areas yearly reports and incidental bulletins are the prime source for government activity. After the war, when MCWA became the CDC, the *CDC Bulletin* assumed this role.

Several books were particularly influential for this project, serving as clear windows into malaria in their place and time. For the nineteenth century, Daniel Drake's writings on malaria played that role: *Malaria in the Interior Valley of North America,* a selection by Norman D. Levine from *A Systematic Treatise, Historical, Etiological, and Practical, of the Principal Diseases of the Interior Valley of North America* . . . (1850; selection published Urbana: University of Illinois Press, 1964). William H. Deaderick and Loyd Thompson, *The Endemic Diseases of the Southern States* (Philadelphia and London: W. B. Saunders, 1916), presented a useful survey of what a southern public health official would have known about malaria and its combat in 1916. Lewis W. Hackett's *Malaria in Europe: An Ecological Study* (London: Oxford University Press, 1937) was particularly valuable in laying out the epidemiology of malaria as understood in the 1930s. A malaria symposium sponsored by the American Association for the Advancement of Science included papers on every aspect of malaria, providing a thorough summary of malariology in 1940: Forest Ray Moulton, ed., *A Symposium on Human Malaria with Special Reference to North America and the Caribbean Region* (Washington, D.C.: AAAS, 1941).

A final word on my approach to historical epidemiology is in order here. For the past twenty to thirty years, historians of medicine have struggled to find ways to describe the ways in which diseases are created and/or found in society and nature. The term "social construction" has been used to indicate the degree to which disease labels are manufactured to meet social needs or address social anxieties. Other scholars use the phrase "framing" to discuss the various factors, biological and social, that put borders around symptom complexes and turn them into disease entities. While there is no denying that cultural factors influence perceptions of and reactions to diseases, there is also no denying that the plasmodium is a real creature, and if it is a new occupant of your body, you are likely to feel very ill indeed. Throughout this study I have taken the biological reality of malaria as a given, while at the same time being sensitive to its changing meanings in society. This seems to me the only reasonable way to write the history of disease. The best discussion of the subtleties of historical disease definition is Charles E. Rosenberg, "Framing Disease," in Rosenberg and Janet Golden, eds., *Framing Disease: Studies in Cultural History* (New Brunswick, N.J.: Rutgers University Press, 1992): xiii–xxvi.

# Index

Note: Italicized page numbers indicate illustrations. Tables are indicated by an italicized *t* following the page number.

charms, 122
Chesapeake area, 25–26
"chills," 134–35
chill tonic, 57, 135
chloroquine, 73, 146
cholera, 42, 43
chronic malaria, 9–10
cinchona bark, 27, 36, 37–38
Civil War, 37–38, 44
Civil Works Administration, 100
climatic influences, 10–12, 152–53
Coclanis, Peter, 25
communication, between physician and
    patient, 117–20
Conecuh River, 90
conjure doctors, 120, 121–24
control outlook, 1
Coolidge, Calvin, 95, 104
Cooper River, 106
Coosa River, 90
cotton farming, 52, 80
Curtin, Philip, 27–28, 68, 73

dams: in Tennessee Valley Authority, 104–5;
    and water impounding, 87–92
DDT: advent of, 147; anopheles mosquito's
    resistance to, 151; campaign of 1940s, 2,
    148–49; in Pacific theater, 142, 147; public
    clamor for, 147–48; and reputation of Cen-
    ters for Disease Control, 140–41; Santee-
    Cooper area as testing grounds, 108; in
    Tennessee Valley Authority, 105; toxicity
    of, 147; World Health Organization cam-
    paigns, 150–51
Deeks, W. E., 78
degeneracy, 59, 63–64
denial, 86–87
diagnostic inaccuracies, 97–98
Dickens, Charles, 31–33, 35
dieldrin, 151
diet and poverty, 126
diphtheria, 61, 69
disease: classification specificity, 42; cultural
    explanations of, 117–20, 139; Drake study,
    34–35; germ theory of, 40, 45–46; higher
    rates among blacks, 59–60; studying
    blacks and, 16; theory from prior cen-
    turies, 119–20
disease etiology: revolution in, 45–48;
    specificity of, 42
disease vector. *See also* anopheles mosqui-
    toes: attacking, 3; first accurate knowledge
    of, 2, 46
Dowling, Oscar, 60, 131–32

Drake, Daniel, 34–35
Duffy antigen, 18, 66, 152
Duke Power Company, 87, 91

Earle, Carville, 24
ecology of malaria, 50–52
economic losses, 83–84
economics, of public health reform, 3–4
educational projects, 81, 87, 133–34
Ehrlich, Paul, 65, 69
*Eingeboren* theory, 46–47
Electric Mills, Mississippi, 84
el Niño, 12
Engber, Barry, 109
epidemics: Connecticut River valley, 38;
    New York City, 38
epidemics, suspected: during Arapaho and
    Cheyenne resettlements, 22–23; Arkansas
    territory, 1819, 22; Jamestown, 17th cen-
    tury, 24; West Coast, 1829–1834, 21–22
eugenics, 59
Ewald, Paul, 14
Ezdorf, R. H. von, 74

Faget, J. C., 44
*falciparum*: acquired immunity to, 19; in
    Africa and South Asia, 152; arrival in New
    World, 23–25; biology of, 8–10, 11–12; in
    Drake study, 34–35; evolutionary history
    of, 13–14; in malariatherapy, 66–67; in San-
    tee-Cooper area, 108; seasons in South,
    70; sickle-cell-trait immunity, 18; yellow
    fever comparison, 43
Faust, Ernest Carroll, 12, 95, 96, 141
Federal Emergency Relief Administration,
    99–100
Federal Power Commission, 89, 90
Federal Writers' Project, 5, 100, 114–17, 123
fetal hemoglobin, 18
Feudtner, Christopher, 113
fever: early medical beliefs, 42; intermittent
    fever, 28; patterns of, 9
"fever and ague" description, 26
Flit, 56, *58*
folk knowledge, 6
Ford, Henry, 104
Freeborn, Stanley, 143, 145
Freeman, Lucian, 124
frontier life, 30–36
fungal spore theories, 42–43

gametocytes, 10, 51, 78
geography, and medical care, 126–27
Goldberger, Joseph, 71–72

debate surrounding, 76–79; dependency on patient cooperation, 77–78; as diagnostic aid, 97; Koch and, 47; limitations of, 39, 57; other uses of, 36; shortages in WWII, 142; side effects of, 76; U.S. Public Health Service promotion, *137*, 139
quinine sterilization, 75–77

race: as barrier to health care, 127; as definable biological variable, 15; as dominant topic, 3; and immunity, 17–20, 46–47; and malaria, 57, 59–62; research dilemmas of, 15–17
racism, 59, 111
railroads, malaria work, 84–85
rainfall, 11–12
Ramsay, David, 30–31
Reed, Walter, 47–48, 69, 72
regional considerations, 24–25, 27–28
religious belief and healing, 121
relocation, as remedy, 27, 108
Revolutionary War soldiers, 28–29
Rice, J. B., 50
River Falls Power Company, 90
rivers, federal regulation of, 88–90
Roanoke Rapids project, 84
Rockefeller Foundation, 71, 74–76, 95
Rocky Mountains, 34
Roosevelt, Franklin, 5, 70, 99, 104
root doctors, 122
Rose, Wickliffe, 74
Ross, Ronald, 6, 46, 69, 72
Rothman, Sheila, 113
rural perceptions, 134–39
Russell, Paul, 56, 142, 149, 151, 153–54
Rutman, Anita, 25–26
Rutman, Darrett, 25–26

salvarsan, 65, 69
sanitation, 37, 45, 132–33
Santee-Cooper Reservoir, 92, 106–8, 146
Santee River, 106
Sappington, John, 36
Sappington's Anti-Fever Pills, 36
screening programs, 80–82
screens, 56
seasonal influences, 11
segregation of infected, 73, 79
*Shadow of the Plantation* (Johnson), 115
sickle-cell hemoglobin, 18, 66–67
Sinclair, Upton, 69
slavery, arguments to justify, 67
smallpox, 37, 42
Social Security Act, 100

socioeconomic factors, 54, 64, 79–80
South: economy and malaria, 52, 54–57; hospitable to breeding, 51–52; malaria comeback in 1930s, 95; malaria control in, 72–82; malaria's retreat to, 38–40; outmigration from countryside, 111–12, 115; parasite rates among blacks, 62, 63*t;* public health activity, 70–72; race and malaria, 57, 59–62
South Carolina, 24–25, 30–31, 106
Southern Farmer's Burden (cartoon), *53*
spell casting, 122
"standard" quinine regimen, 75–77
Stannard, David, 21
streams, federal regulation of, 88–90
superstitions, 116
suspicion: in antimosquito work, 132; of physicians, 129–30
swamps: association with malaria, 26, 31; in Dickens's fiction, 32; Drake's observations, 34; medical knowledge about, 40; New Deal drainage projects, 99–103
Sydenham, Thomas, 26
symptoms, 9–10
syphilis, 16, 65–67, 69, 116

Tennessee River, 103–6
Tennessee Valley Authority (TVA), 88, 92, 103–6
Thermaline, 36
Thomas, Elbert, 143
toilets, 132–33
Tommasi-Crudeli, Corrado, 45
training film, 142
tuberculosis: among American blacks, 15, 16, 60–61; carriers of, 61; control of, 69; degeneracy argument, 64
Tuskegee syphilis study, 16, 118, 130
TVA (Tennessee Valley Authority), 88, 92, 103–6
Twain, Mark, 33
typhoid fever, 45, 61
Typhoid Mary, 61, 65
typhomalaria, 44–45

underdeveloped nations, 150
Underwood, F. J., 86
United States, currently imported cases, 1–2
upper Mississippi valley, 38–40
U.S. Public Health Service: budget cuts, 95, 99; DDT campaign of 1940s, 2; emergency funds for, 100; malaria control efforts, 74–76; merchant studies, 83–84; reorganization of, 143; survey of Santee-Cooper area, 107–8; against yellow fever, 69